The Natural State of Medical Practice

Implications

Volume IV

William H. Adams, M.D.

LIBERTY HILL PUBLISHING

Liberty Hill Publishing
2301 Lucien Way #415
Maitland, FL 32751
407.339.4217
www.libertyhillpublishing.com

Paperback ISBN-13: 978-1-66287-084-2
Hard Cover ISBN-13: 978-1-66287-085-9

For Diana, Judith and Beth,
with gratitude for their
advice and support

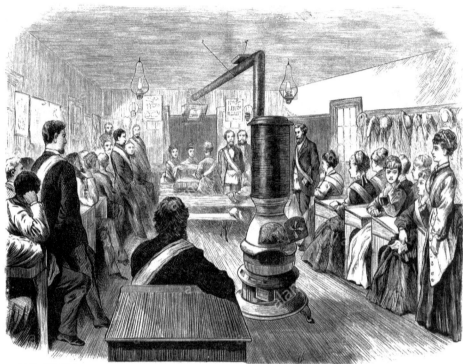

ILLINOIS.—THE GRANGE MOVEMENT—THE LODGE-ROOM IN THE SCHOOLHOUSE NEAR EDWARDSVILLE DURING THE SESSION OF THE LOCAL GRANGE.—SKETCHED BY OUR SPECIAL ARTIST. JOSEPH E. BEALE.

In addition to the essential role of natural rights of the individual as prominently discussed in this volume, it is the work of associations of individuals seeking self-betterment that is essential to initiation and promotion of human progress. One such association was a Greek association, the koinon (κοινων), which *The Natural State of Medical Practice* poses as the collegial affiliation that led to ancient Hippocratic medicine. Pictured here is a different 19th C association, a Grange meeting where community plans and issues were deliberated. Alexis de Tocqueville carefully described the multiplicity of local associations as a uniquely American phenomenon (see Excursus 15, p. 153). He also stated that the greater the equality in a society the greater should be the number and role of associations.

THE NATURAL STATE OF MEDICAL PRACTICE: IMPLICATIONS

MONOGRAPHS EXAMINING IN DETAIL SELECT ISSUES PRESENTED IN PRECEDING VOLUMES OF THE *NATURAL STATE OF MEDICAL PRACTICE*

By
William H. Adams, MD

The front cover is a popular illustration of the Ten Commandments (the Decalogue) in Paleo-Hebrew (used as early as 1000 BC) and considered a restatement of natural law. It was chosen to display the common element of Judeo-Christianity that explains the appearance in the West of modern medical practice, a doubling of human longevity, moral abolition of slavery, and the negative effects of disregarding them. Much of this volume describes the mechanisms by which that common element has been and is being disregarded and the consequences thereof.

PREFACE

The rapid expansion in human knowledge and the scale of its effects occasioned by technology are arousing revolutionary opinions regarding the future of mankind and questioning the relevance of its past. But *The Natural State of Medical Practice* and its social history of medical practice has demonstrated that the nature of responses by societies to dramatic events over thousands of years, events that occurred under a wide range of circumstances, human and environmental, have remained remarkably consistent. They are, therefore, predictable. Surprisingly, the nature of the responses is not complex as long as we do not get caught up analyzing the tangled myriad of particulars, personages, philosophies and prejudices involved. And so, using medical practice and human longevity as a gauge of progress, it is from seeing the forest rather than just the trees that the following political conclusions have been derived:

1. A "natural state" of medical practice, the only status capable of medical progress, is possible only in a free society.
2. The freedom of that society must include civil liberty based on natural rights and natural law.
3. Our civilization, recognizing natural rights and natural law, is the only true mature civilization that has existed on earth and is the source of all progress.
4. Our civilization is Judeo-Christian, for its common thread and the source of its success is natural law/Decalogue.
5. All progress is the product of the common man and woman, the unprivileged citizenry of a civilization, and occurs when their natural rights are protected.
6. Government by its very nature is a locus of incompetence and has never been the source of progress in any form.
7. Big government is the forest.

In reaching these conclusions, among many others, *The Natural State of Medical Practice* and the enclosed series of related excursus dismissively characterize many human agencies and institutions throughout history and prehistory as not contributing to human progress. These include:

1. "Great" civilizations of Mesopotamia, Egypt, China, India, and Greco-Roman
2. Traditional "medicine," including shamanism, exorcist-priests, Ayurveda, and Traditional Chinese Medicine
3. Most of the world's atheists and religions, except for Judeo-Christianity
4. Modern health care, increasingly including aspects of our own
5. The political elite classes and their abettors and beneficiaries
6. Governments, authoritarian or egalitarian (which is *per ipsum* authoritarian)

Thus, in addition to our contemporary proselytizers of a New Age and deniers of the Old, the populations of the Near and Middle East, Asia, and many in the West, sympathizers and practitioners of alternative medicine, religious populations other than Judeo-Christian, governments other than those based on natural law and natural rights, and most contemporary politicians, medical practitioners, and academics in sociology, archeology, anthropology, classical studies, political science, and history/prehistory will view my work as idiosyncratic, biased, wrong, or simply naive. This leaves virtually no one left who, as I relate in Excursus 12, can see the forest for the trees. This is unfortunate, for the conclusions of *The Natural State of Medical Practice* are correct. Read for yourself.

William H. Adams, MD
Hobart, New York
January, 2023

VOLUME 4
CONTENTS

The following is a summary of volumes 1 and 3 of *The Natural State of Medical Practice* (Maitland, FL, 2019). An abridgement has been published, *Medical Practice and the Common Man and Woman: A History*, but at seven hundred pages an even more brief version has been requested, but one that includes all major salient points the unabridged work encompasses. That approach is presented here, roughly approximating the sequence as found in the abridgement's thirty-eight chapters (and accordingly bracketed in bold { } for ready reference to the abridgement's chapters), with the understanding that much evidence supporting the work's conclusions is to be found only in the unabridged volumes.[1]

This excursus, a summary of the political implications of *The Natural State of Medical Practice*, is an "opening salvo" for much that follows. It identifies the role of descriptive science, or "inductive" reasoning, in the work's conclusions, the relevance of human freedom to natural law, and, supported by statistical proof, the essential role of the unprivileged but free "common man and woman" to human progress as gauged by life expectancy. The conclusion targets modern threats to progress.

By interpreting natural law as a statement on the inviolability of human liberty, identification of infractions of natural law become less subjective. In this excursus a proof is offered that identifies natural law as purposeful and beneficial because both increased life expectancy and an effective collegial medical association are shown to be products of human liberty. In effect, it directs us toward a secular Eden. It is also confirmed that natural law is an attribute of all mankind and unrelated to race, ethnicity, unique characteristics, or social class. It concludes with the observation that natural law in secular governance in the West, despite its limited extent and whether intended or not, has spread the beneficence of natural law globally. The tragic consequences should it be lost are predicted.

---

[1] Volume 2, *The Natural State of Medical Practice: Hippocratic Evidence*, is primarily a translation of several important Hippocratic treatises presented in a relatively literal interlinear format followed by a vernacular translation. Its value to this trilogy is that its new translations support the conclusions concerning the prominence of ancient Greek medicine referred to in the other two volumes.

The philosophical orientation of this excursus is an attempt to bypass the many versions and definitions of virtue over the ages and to assign to natural law that which is its due, namely the source of the freedom that permits virtue. Based on *The Natural State of Medical Practice*, it then develops a theorem: *Human progress and true virtue, as expressions of natural law, can occur only in a free society*, refers to its supporting evidence, and places its significance in today's world.

That the universe is not "unfolding as it should" is the topic of this excursus, for the history of the world is the history of the consequences of authoritarianism. There have been a few brief periods when this was not so, and supporting evidence from the history of medical practice is briefly repeated. It was, however, the post-Reformation West that saw a broad and sustained release of the ingenuity of the unprivileged population (common citizenry). This, plus a reaffirmation of the democratic alliance of physician and patient, first clearly expressed by Hippocratic physicians, brought about the profusion of medical knowledge that has led to a striking increase in life expectancy, first in the West and then globally. But the history of medical practice also clearly demonstrates the calamitous sequels to political interference, such as is occurring today. Predictable consequences to modern medicine are detailed.

The common identity of natural law, the Decalogue and the Golden Rule is argued in this excursus, and a common interpretation is derived: Do not transgress the rights of others. An explanation for the tardy mindfulness of natural law and natural rights by mankind is offered, and the scope of their authority is extended to include government itself. It is argued that in brief periods in early urbanization before powerful political hierarchies had yet to transgress natural law there was evidence of progress in medicine, but transgression promptly intervened, and progress ceased. This changed with the 16th C Reformation because natural law and natural rights were increasingly acknowledged and, into the 17th C, natural rights were increasingly protected. Consequently, the 18th C saw the emergence of medical discovery that flourished in the 19th C, and the 20th C saw the West as the intellectual center of the world. Such was the power of complying with natural law.

A description of mankind's natural aversion to crowding as displayed by primitive nomadic and sedentary groups opens this excursus. Manifested in small groups by early humans for social contact and protections centering around family, it is proposed that larger and thereby more authoritarian kinships were preferentially avoided except for safety. In rare but remarkable instances the repressive early tribal kinship was abandoned for commercial urbanization, although ensuing progress would, within a few centuries, be blocked by authoritarian political governance. This is a warning that the ethic of natural law encounters increasing risk of subversion as population density increases and we lose or cede our natural rights and responsibilities to a politicized central governance. Should this occur the consequence will be perennial conflict and regression of progress already obtained. Would that it were possible to safely disperse.

This excursus reviews human progress as a consequence of liberty of the unprivileged, or common, man and woman, and integrates the ancient Hebraic ethos into that sequence. Most religions do not weigh liberty of the individual as a doctrinal element and have not been associated with secular progress. In contrast, the Judeo-Christian religion from the beginning has, in recognizing all people as descendants of God's original creation and therefore of equal importance to God, retained an egalitarian sympathy for human liberty. There were several transient expressions of civil liberty resulting in medical progress in the ancient world. But it was only with the Reformation that there occurred a transposition of that Judaic egalitarian sympathy to governance in the West, the result being two-and-a-half centuries of human progress that have immeasurably improved the lives of billions around the world. This is the first time in human history that civil liberty, the offspring of the ancient Hebrew acknowledgement of the equal status of every individual before God, has been purposely sanctioned and ultimately codified within a civilization, and its astounding success argues it should become both permanent and global.

Epidemiological data extracted from the anthropological and archeological literature of early humans and from other hominids as reviewed here are inconsistent with the argument that *Homo sapiens* is a product of evolution on earth.

Epidemiological proofs presented in *The Natural State of Medical Practice* support the Isagorial Theory of Human Progress. They also (1) support core tenets of Objectivist philosophy and (2) support the concept of natural law. Furthermore, the morality of Objectivism is consistent with that of Judeo-Christianity. Despite its refutation of religion or any intellectual discipline based on faith, the limitations of this Objectivist stance are reviewed and a justification for mutual accommodation is presented. For Objectivism it is central to its philosophy that individuals do not transgress on another's life. In Isagorial Theory that principle is acknowledged to be ancient and cosmopolitan (Judeo-Christian) and active today via the human conscience (natural law). But Isagorial Theory does more than identify the evils of transgression on others. It identifies the primary problem, which is not the individual. It is, instead, authoritarian governance by a political elite. When that authoritarianism is blocked, civil liberty will lead to success of the entrepreneurial group and the community as a whole will benefit. Replace authoritarian governance and there will be little need for philosophy-derived correctives.

This is an explanatory monograph on the purpose and significance of the message presented on the **contratyrannos.com** website of the Isagorial Theory of Human Progress. That theory, derived from *The Natural State of Medical Practice*, is not about herbal therapies, alternative medicine, or the beauties of primitivism. It does not promote any inherent ethnic or geographic superiority in advancing human progress. Nor, in its references to the "common man and woman," is it an attempt to instigate a rebellion among the disadvantaged. It is, instead, a warning to everyone of danger to human progress that lies ahead, a warning exposed by this social history of medical practice as interpreted by a physician.

Following a formal validation of Isagorial Theory, the unintended consequences of authoritarian interference in society's natural rights are shown to reside in big government, thus giving us the warning:

> From him who sees no wood for trees,
> And yet is busie as the bees
> From him that's settled on his lees
> And speaketh not without his fees,
> Libera nos.

An important question regarding the disappearance from five ancient civilizations of early attempts at developing a rational medical profession is why, once they disappeared, there was no further attempt to initiate another. The delayed commencement of modern medicine is a story of enormous consequence, and, after a brief review of the ancient losses, causes of the delay are considered. Two reasons seem most likely, both attributable to an all-powerful political hierarchy: canonization of venerable medical knowledge resistant to change and marginalization of the common citizenry from whom the original rational medical knowledge arose.

In this excursus the novel declaration is made and argued that our present "Western" civilization is the only true civilization in human history.

Human progress, which Excursus 14 argued is a necessary component of the definition of a civilization, was proposed in *The Natural State of Medical Practice* to emerge in early societies from individuals collaborating in common council to improve their condition in life. Through such collaborative groups ideas can be improved and vetted to the benefit of the members and, when applied to society, can lead to improvement in the lives of everyone. Thus, whenever the government restricts the natural exploitation of ingenuity for self-betterment, government not only limits an individual's options for his or her personal well-being. It also blocks the benefits that can emerge from a new idea or discovery being introduced into society. Also in this excursus, human ingenuity (as a facet of human reason) is postulated as a counterpart to natural law. Natural law is our protection against other humans, but ingenuity is our protection against everything else. I propose that purposeful limitations by government on one's attempt at improving, by legal means, one's condition in life can be considered equivalent to violation of natural law. It is detrimental to both the individual and society, even to its survival.

An analysis of our present civilization, often identified as "Western," affirms the importance of the Reformation as its source. The Reformation was preceded by a thousand years without progress in the West, at least in medicine, and therefore was a period classifiable more as a culture than a civilization. But the catalyst of the Reformation exposed the Decalogue as an ethical guide not just for individuals but for governance as well, and it is the latter that has led to Western progress and the Constitution and Bill of Rights of the United States. The Decalogue, transmitted to the ancient Israelites, brought to the fore the primary requirements for a progressive civilization, but demography did not provide the ancient Israelites with the opportunity to formally establish a civilization. This was remedied in the post-Reformation West when Jewish and Christian contributions to civil liberties made it possible to instill progress into our own society. Mosaic history thereby became part of our own. It is concluded that there has been only one true mature civilization, the Judeo-Christian civilization. Its global recognition and replication augur well for mankind's future if the Decalogue continues to guide both the individual and the State.

Excursus 17 – Physicians or Pharaoh's Priests 177

In an effort to unite the history of medical practice with events and portents of the present day, the appearance and disappearance of rational medicine in ancient civilizations is again reviewed. Focus is on the practitioner over the ages, how medical progress emerged solely from the clinical efforts of the practitioner, and how interference in the practitioner's domain profoundly inhibited medical progress. The mechanisms of that interference are summarized and then shown to be similar to recent events in American medicine. It is concluded that medicine is increasingly under the control of an authoritarian political class, and that intrusion into the physician-patient relation will turn our profession into a trade and restrict clinical progress. Government, *per se*, has never contributed to human progress, but in America constitutional safeguards have protected our natural rights by limiting the role of government. This is being dangerously undermined.

Excursus 18 -The Reformation, Enslavement, and the Isagorial Theory of Human Progress 209

We are all descendants of both slaves and enslavers. In its briefest terms, this excursus acknowledges enslavement as a normal component of all past civilizations. At the same time, natural law makes clear to every person that enslavement is immoral. The explanation for this seeming paradox is that natural law has been overruled by positive (man-made) laws and actions imposed by authoritarian dictate. The Ten Commandments (the Decalogue) are a formal exposition of natural law expressed in Judeo-Christian scripture, and they affirmed the abnegation of slavery to the West. Yet enslavement persisted. But the Reformation then declared the equal status of all persons before God, following which secular leadership and citizens began to be viewed as equals and equally subject to natural law. As legislatures became more representative of their citizens, natural law was increasingly incorporated into secular laws defending natural rights. Remarkably, just as it took two-and-a-half centuries after the onset of the Reformation for modern medical progress to appear, the same period was required for abolitionism to be initiated on a national scale. Morality and ingenuity of the common citizenry were unleashed simultaneously. Such is the power of associations of a free people when endowed with natural rights and guided by natural law instead of authoritarian governance run by a privileged political class. The abolition of slavery, like medical progress, can thus be explained by the *Isagorial Theory of Human Progress*, which now seems to encompass the political as well as apolitical betterment of mankind.[2] Although the preceding is a Western drama unique in the history of civilizations, the Judeo-Christian Decalogue, as a formal statement of natural law, is the birthright of all humanity.

---

[2] Definition of *Isagorial Theory of Human Progress*: A theory ascribing all apolitical advances for the betterment of mankind to autonomous associations pursuing self-betterment in which each member has equal opportunity to speak freely and share ideas about the group's common interest without fear of retribution. Axiomatically it excludes "betterments" that have been stolen, copied, derived by exploitation, or used for subjugation of others. (See Excursus 12, Validation of the Isagorial Theory of Human Progress.)

LOCATION OF SOME NOTABLE CONCLUSIONS IN THE FIRST THREE VOLUMES OF *THE NATURAL STATE OF MEDICAL PRACTICE*

It is likely that *The Natural State of Medical Practice,* in four volumes, will be read in its completeness by few people. It is long and covers facets of many academic disciplines, each of which can rightfully claim its own brace of superior experts. Why spend time on a physician's amalgamation of expert opinion in areas beyond his expertise, especially as the author declares it to be a proof that the Judeo-Christian civilization is the only mature civilization to ever have existed, and, since the Reformation, the source of modern global progress. Even though he claims *The Natural State of Medical Practice* contains supporting proof for his *Isagorial Theory of Human Progress*, its seemingly obvious and biased implausibility will in itself deter many a reader.

For convenience to the curious, however, the following list identifies the major topics of this volume, and, in the second list, locates major conclusions in relevant chapters of the first three volumes of *The Natural State of Medical Practice*. This should make it easier for the reader to quickly evaluate the evidence about a topic of interest. Once immersed in that, perhaps curiosity about the bigger picture presented in *The Natural State of Medical Practice* will lead the reader to seek a greater exposure to its contents.

I. List of the present volume's Excursus topics in a word:

Excursus 1 – Summary
Excursus 2 – Focus
Excursus 3 – Natural law
Excursus 4 – Morality and virtue
Excursus 5 – Historicism
Excursus 6 – The Decalogue
Excursus 7 – Judeo-Christianity
Excursus 8 – Natural rights
Excursus 9 – Evolution
Excursus 10 – Objectivism
Excursus 11 – Authoritarianism
Excursus 12 – Isagorial theory
Excursus 13 – Common people
Excursus 14 – Civilization defined
Excursus 15 – Ingenuity
Excursus 16 – Judeo-Christian civilization
Excursus 17 – Canonization and Corporatism
Excursus 18 – Slavery

15

II. Notable conclusions and location of their principal arguments, most by the first page of the relevant chapter:

Volume 1 – The Natural State of Medical Practice: An Isagorial Theory of Human Progress

Volume 2 – The Natural State of Medical Practice: Hippocratic Evidence

Volume 3 – The Natural State of Medical Practice: Escape from Egalitarianism

DEFINITIONS

1. Authoritarianism: unconditional coercive social control at the expense of personal freedom.
2. City-state: an autonomous or self-sufficient state consisting of a central city and its surrounding interdependent smaller settlements.
3. Civilization: an autonomous and self-sufficient urban and rural population sufficiently large to produce a surplus of food for trade that contributes to wealth and permits specialization of crafts and vocations to the benefit of.[3]
4. Corporatism: (1) primitive society - central control of construction and production by special interest groups; (2) complex society – "a system of interest intermediation linking producer interests and the state, in which explicitly recognized interest organizations are incorporated into the policy-making process ..." (Oxford Concise Dictionary).
5. Egalitarian kinship: a consanguineal and affinal group in which assigned status implements opinions and traditions regarding redistribution of effort.
6. Egalitarian: archeologically defined, in whole or in part, as a society with no differential wealth in burials, dwellings, districts, or architecture, and no monumental structures, militarization or a distinct long-lived population.
7. Egalitarianism (social or coercive): an authoritarian doctrine that would forcibly interfere with voluntary choice by imposing social or economic equality or equity on a society.
8. Group: "a number of individuals having some unifying relationship." (Merriam-Webster; and see "koinon" below.)
9. Heterarchy: a multifocal system of management in a social system in which there is no permanent head.
10. Historicism: a theory in which history is seen as a determinant of events, past and future.
11. Individualism: advocating or tolerating political and economic independence of the individual.
12. Isagorial Theory of Human Progress: a theory ascribing all apolitical advances for the betterment of mankind to autonomous associations pursuing self-betterment in which each member has equal opportunity to speak freely and share ideas about the group's common interest without fear of retribution. Axiomatically it excludes "betterments" that have been stolen, copied, derived by exploitation, or used for subjugation of others. (See "koinon".)
13. Kinship: a universal form of social organization based on a real or alleged culturally defined family ties and rules of behavior.

---

[3] This definition assumes that storage contributes to accumulation of wealth. It is a minimalist definition because the object of this volume is an analysis of the earliest stages of urbanization rather than urbanization in full flower. It differs from the definition used in volume 1 because a tiered governing hierarchy is not specifically identified, but it is implied in the "settlement hierarchy" mentioned herein in the five "successful" civilizations. It is also somewhat at variance with that of Dr. B. G. Trigger (*Understanding Early Civilizations*, Cambridge, 2003, p. 46) who defined early civilizations as the "earliest and simplest form of *class-based* society." Social classes may have been a consequence of commercial success but not their cause or goal.

14. Koinon: an autonomous voluntary and democratic group sharing a common self-interest that meets in common council to freely exchange information and experiences pertinent to all its members.
15. Natural law: a body of unchanging moral principles regarded as a basis for all human conduct (Oxford English Dictionary).
16. Natural rights: the general right of individuals to life, liberty, property and pursuit of happiness, rights considered inherent, universal, and "do not arise out of any special relationship or transaction between men."[4]
17. Objectivism: the concept of man as a heroic being, with his own happiness as the moral purpose of his life (Ayn Rand). Merriam-Webster states: "any of various theories asserting the validity of objective phenomena over subjective experience."[5]
18. Primary city or city-state: an early city-state that is not a colony and is unaffiliated with a larger civilization.
19. Primary civilization: a civilization that has not been "shaped by substantial dependence upon or control by other, more complex societies."[6]
20. Progress: for a society, a social concept based on the awareness of improvability of the human condition.
21. Settlement hierarchy: intergroup adjustments that spontaneously occur as a virgin urbanizing society, unaffiliated with a larger civilization and having no prior experience with a political hierarchy, becomes more complex and acquires facilities, goods and services to accommodate an enlarging population.
22. Virtue: moral excellence.

---

[4] Some of this definition is from: Hart, H. L. A., *Are There Any Natural Rights?*, in *The Philosophical Review*, 64:175-191, 1955. Issues related to legal implications of competing "rights" are irrelevant here.

[5] Merriam-Webster, definition (1).

[6] Trigger, B. G., *Understanding Early Civilizations*, Cambridge, 2003, p. 19.

INTRODUCTION

The eighteen excursus[7] in this volume expand on themes presented in the three volumes of *The Natural State of Medical Practice*. Each volume also has its own internal series of excursus relevant to its purpose, and the present series, while separate, builds on all three.

To assist the reader in integrating the broad and at times tedious repetition and frequently overlapping range of topics and definitions covered in *The Natural State of Medical Practice* and in the excursus of this volume, an austere summary of its interlocking ideas is presented below. Its unexpected deviations from standard historical interpretation will seem for some readers to be disconnected from the facts. For this reason, the related sections in the first three volumes of *The Natural State of Medical Practice* are frequently referenced throughout the eighteen excursus so that the supporting arguments and references can be readily accessed. I have stated elsewhere that I am not a historian, an anthropologist, archeologist or sociologist. Thus, my arguments, such as are based on fact and knowledgeable opinion, are based on the facts and interpretations of experts in those fields as expressed in textbooks and scientific publications. It is only their juxtaposition in the history of human progress that I can declare as my own work, and even that is limited. For medical issues I can claim more credit.

We begin with an acknowledgement of inadequacies in modern medical practice, as that was my instigation for seeking ideas from other times and civilizations that might improve our own medical care. It became quickly apparent, however, that the issues were social rather than medical. The history of ancient Greek medicine was especially susceptible to understanding because I translated a number of Hippocratic treatises from the Greek. Their clinical expertise was readily apparent. Why did Hippocratic medicine not continue to progress? How could it happen that for a thousand years through the European Dark Ages and Medieval Period rational and scientific medicine was consigned to oblivion? Then, on studying ancient Egyptian medicine it was immediately obvious that there was undoubted clinical expertise described in Papyrus Ebers, but knowledge in the available copy from 1550 BC was never amended or improved and, but for some limited copying, had all but disappeared fifteen hundred years later. Furthermore, that 1550 BC Papyrus Ebers claims to have been originally composed in the 1st Dynasty, another fifteen hundred years earlier, clear evidence of lack of progress over that extensive period. As a skeptical novice with these seemingly bizarre and unexpected but factual bits of history of medical practice and impressed by the chronologic extremes to which entire civilizations could be condemned to utter medical ignorance, an examination of other civilizations seemed necessary, and a precis of that search is now presented:

MEDICAL PROGRESS: A TRIUMPH OF THE JUDEO-CHRISTIAN CIVILIZATION

When did the concept of medical progress first appear? Ever since the first man and woman, disease, trauma and an early grave have been mankind's lot. Motivation to prevent, treat or delay them is common to all members of our species, rich or poor, ever

---

[7] The plural of the Latin *excursus*, a 4th declension noun, is *excursus*, with the second *u* being long in the latter, short in the former. In English the plural of "excursus" is also excursus.

since biblical Adam and Eve (or the popular Y-chromosomal Adam and Mitochondrial Eve).

The first clear evidence of medical progress is found in early medical writings of five ancient civilizations (regionally identified as Mesopotamian, Egyptian, Indian, Chinese, and ancient Greece), and the social environment at the time their clinical wisdom was collected is consistent with early primary urbanization, usually the "settlement hierarchy" stage, defined as intergroup adjustments that spontaneously occur as a virgin urbanizing society, unaffiliated with a larger civilization and **having no prior experience with a political hierarchy**, becomes more complex and acquires facilities, goods and services to accommodate an enlarging population.[8]

Unfortunately, the "spontaneous" freedoms of the settlement hierarchy stage were not followed by social evolution into free and democratic civilizations. Instead, the commercially guided and relatively egalitarian early primary city-states were replaced by sequential totalitarian dynasties in Mesopotamia, Egypt, and China, by scattered monarchical rule in India (following decline of the Indus River Valley Civilization), and by authoritarian wars that destroyed the civilization of ancient Greece.

Once monarchical political power was imposed in the five historical civilizations all medical progress permanently ceased, sometimes disappearing altogether, and much or all of the population of the cited civilizations returned to a baseline level of empirical medical knowledge. In those instances where ancient medical wisdom persisted, it was canonized by the ruling political hierarchy and became impervious to change. The cause of *failure to progress*, the subject of volume 1, was now apparent: authoritarian political governance.

The possibility that early medical progress had occurred in lesser-known large societies or civilizations was minimized by analyzing data from twelve prehistorical civilizations around the world. None had evidence of medical professionals.[9] Why?

All seventeen historical and prehistorical civilizations/societies were then analyzed as a group, the purpose being to detect those characteristics that permitted a civilization to initiate medical progress. It was concluded in volume 3 that, statistically, the most likely cause for *failure to initiate* medical progress was the authoritarianism of the kinship associated with tribal or clan loyalties and obligations.

Noting that the common feature of a civilization's failure to initiate or to improve a medical practice was centralized authoritarian political power, our own civilization was then examined for the same parameters. The following sequence describes its unique course:

(16th C) The release of much of the European population from feudalism and the super-kinship that had been led by the Roman Catholic Church for a thousand years

---

[8] The ancient medical writings, their civilizations, and my estimates for dates of their original data collection are:
1. *Treatise of Medical Diagnosis and Prognosis* (Mesopotamian/Sumer, *ca.* 3000 BC)
2. *Papyrus Ebers* (originally composed *ca.* 3000 BC, the time of Egyptian unification)
3. The *Charaka Samhita* (The Collection of Charaka) (India, *ca.* 2000 BC)
4. The *Huang Ti Nei Ching Su Wen* (The Yellow Emperor's Classic of Internal Medicine) (China, *ca.* 2400 BC)
5. The *Corpus Hippocraticum* (Greece, *ca.* 5th century BC)

[9] The civilizations/city-states analyzed were: Marajoara, Norte Chico (Caral Supe), Poverty Point, Cahokia, Terramare, Catalhoyuk, Djenne-Djenno, Sintashta, Shahr-i Sokhta, Liangzhou, Anasazi (Chaco Canyon), and Cucuteni-Trypillian.

followed recognition of the equality of all persons before God, a desire for religious freedom, and a claim that, in effect, the Ten Commandments (the Decalogue, often viewed as natural law or as the basis of common law) should apply to society's leadership and governance as well as to individuals.[10] The subsequent civil liberties of the common citizenry of Western civilization can be traced to the Reformation.

(17th C) Because of the demand for civil freedoms and the concurrent curtailment of Vatican power, parliamentary rule increased in importance and the common citizenry began to pursue commercial self-betterment rather than betterment of their "betters." Another product of expanding civil liberties was the Enlightenment (17th/18th centuries).

(18th C) Natural rights became constitutionally protected and the medical ingenuity of the common citizenry was now discernible.

(19th C) Medical discovery reached its zenith, and life expectancy began increasing markedly for the majority of a civilization for the first time in human history.

(20th C) Globalization of Western progress in medicine ensued and began replacing all other forms of medical care, including the remnants of canonized medical knowledge that still existed in China, the Middle East and India. Life expectancy continued to increase and to spread around the globe.

In summary, freedom from the authoritarian kinship that allowed individuals to pursue commercial interests in ancient early urbanization was mirrored in expanding civil liberties and commercial prosperity of regions of Europe following the Reformation. Remarkably, despite growth in monarchical power in some sectors (*i.e.*, the Age of Absolutism, 17th/18th centuries), the ethical components of the Decalogue were increasingly transformed into constitutional protections for all persons. This was critical. The earlier evolution to an absolute centralized hierarchy of power that hitherto had led all prior civilizations to cease medical progress was itself stopped dead in its tracks.

The message of the Decalogue, after more than three thousand years, had finally been properly heeded beyond its Hebraic home and to varying degrees had become legislated. Western progress, which is now global progress and which has raised the life expectancy of the common man and woman from 30-40 years to 80 years within the past two centuries, has been one triumphal result.

But what of the 21st C? As common citizenry cede ever more power and personal freedom to a centralized political hierarchy in return for transient benefits now and economic serfdom for imminent generations, as we see wide-ranging canonization of moral and political views and regulations in medicine that conveniently represent government preferment and severely trespass on the doctor-patient relation, the future of medicine, or, at the very least, medical progress, is in great jeopardy. We are reverting to

---

[10] The ethical Commandments are, from the Septuagint:

    a.   You will not kill; οὐ φονεύσεις

    b.   You will not commit adultery; οὐ μοιχεύσεις

    c.   You will not rob; οὐ κλέψεις

    d.   You will not bear false witness; οὐ ψευδομαρτυρήσεις κατα τοῦ πλησίον σου μαρτυρίαν ψευδῆ

    e.   You will not lust after your neighbor's wife, house, field, servant, maid, ox, ass, cattle or whatever belongs to your neighbor; οὐκ επιθυμήσεις τὴν γυναῖκα τοῦ πλησίον σου ουκ ἐπιθυμήσεις τὴν οικιαν τοῦ πλψσίον σου ουτε το αγρον αυτου ουτε τον παιδα αυτου ουτε την παιδισκην αυτου ουτε του βοοσ αυτου ουτε του ὑποζυγιου αυτου ουτε παντος κτηνους αυτου ουτε οσα τω πλψσιον σου εστιν

the Age of Absolutism and all that entails. If the present course is not changed and if medical progress is indeed a bellwether for progress in general, difficult times lie ahead for the young.

EXCURSUS 1

The following is a summary of volumes 1 and 3 of *The Natural State of Medical Practice* (Maitland, FL, 2019). An abridgement has been published, *Medical Practice and the Common Man and Woman: A History* (Maitland, FL, 2020) but at seven hundred pages an even more brief version has been requested, but one that includes all major salient points the unabridged work encompasses. That approach is presented here, roughly approximating the sequence as found in the abridgement's thirty-eight chapters (and accordingly bracketed in bold { } for ready reference to the abridgement's chapters), with the understanding that much evidence supporting the work's conclusions is to be found only in the unabridged volumes.[1]

THE NATURAL STATE OF MEDICAL PRACTICE, A SUMMARY [2]

PART I
Historical Assessment

Every person is susceptible to pain, emotional distress and death associated with disease and trauma, and every person is motivated to lessen their effects. To understand *The Natural State of Medical Practice* and to explain the profound conclusions concerning human progress that emerged from its study, we therefore use medical practice as a universal gauge of progress. Thus, first we must analyze the great variety of medical practices that have existed throughout history and prehistory so that characteristics of success and failure at medical progress can be identified.

{1} To begin, there must be mention of the medicine-man or shaman, who some think represents the ancient and primitive forebear of the modern physician. This is incorrect. The method of the medicine-man has been, without exception, devoted to manipulating demons and controlling fellow humans, not disease. The medicine-man, often the possessor of deviant behavioral characteristics, is shown to be the forebear of the psychic and the huckster, and he has no place in the history of medicine. Empirical medicine finds its roots instead in the anxious observations of practical individuals in family units or tribes who sought, without official sanction, remedies for pain and disease for themselves, their families and neighbors.

---

[1] The previous three volumes are:

Vol. 1 – *The Natural State of Medical Practice: An Isagorial Theory of Human Progress.*
Vol. 2 – *The Natural State of Medical Practice: Hippocratic Evidence*
Vol. 3 – *The Natural State of Medical Practice: Escape from Egalitarianism*
Volume 2 is primarily a translation of several important Hippocratic treatises presented in a relatively literal interlinear format followed by a vernacular translation. Its value to this trilogy is that its new translations support the conclusions concerning the prominence of ancient Greek medicine referred to in the other two volumes.

[2] A "natural state of medical practice" is an established, objective (rational) and clinically effective medical practice free from institutional influences or other forms of external coercion except for those interpersonal influences to which both physician and patient are equally exposed and susceptible. It does not include an individual occasionally dispensing nostrums.

{2}   But with increasing regional populations there developed larger societies and, ultimately, great civilizations. Chaos was prevented by authoritarian rule at the highest level and elitist interpretation of custom at lower levels. Mystical or theurgical beliefs accompanied the transformation of the medicine-man to priest, a more predictable form of population control. Thus, the early Mesopotamian civilization of Sumer had acquired by 3000 BC an early form of rational medicine and a primordial physician, the *azu*, although the nature of that medicine and its practitioners is only now being appreciated. Documentation of clinical acuity has been demonstrated in translations of the ancient Babylonian (but in my opinion originally Sumerian) *Treatise of Medical Diagnosis and Prognosis*. But consolidation of individual Sumerian city-states into kingdoms, followed by 2000 years of monarchical empires that included the Babylonian and Assyrian, was associated with domination of the *azu* and his medical practice by the palace favorite, the exorcist-priest, or *asipu*. Mysticism prevailed, and as the Common Era approached any Sumerian rational medicine had, despite Babylonian emendations, ceased to exist.

{3}   Nine hundred miles to the west, ancient Egyptian medicine was developing what would be renowned as the foundation of Western medicine, although enthusiasm for this theory is not unanimous. It is the writings of the predynastic and early dynasties, *ca*. 3000 BC, as revealed in the famous 1550 BC copies known as *Papyrus Ebers* and the Edwin Smith papyrus, that provide insight into empirical and rational medical practices. But, appropriated by the priest-caste of the early pharaonic State, that empirical-rational medicine became manipulated canon. Thus, a mere twelve papyri grace the medicine of a 2500-year-old empire, a component of many of the twelve being but repetitions of clinical cases or sections from the *Papyrus Ebers*, which therefore must be considered the high point of ancient Egyptian medicine (*i.e.*, 5,000 years ago). Despite a promising beginning, medicine in North Africa, just as in Mesopotamia, came to nothing long before the Common Era.

{4}   Looking now to the east, there is a tenuous early historical record for Asian medicine, but the *Huang Ti Nei Ching Su Wen*, assembled in the 2nd C BC, is said to encapsulate ancient Chinese medical thought.[3] Legend, however, proposes the origin of its clinical material to be *ca*. 2500 BC during the formative years of a unifying China under the Longshan culture emperor, Huang Ti. There are undoubtedly valid clinical diagnostics in this document, and, especially important, it is not mystical and it acknowledges the uniqueness of the individual patient. Nevertheless, its theories and treatments reveal a codified system of disease and physiology with no basis in fact, a fabrication rather than a misunderstanding. It is remarkable that a civilization known for its many manifestations of brilliance would validate such a basis for medical practice, but the fault can be traced to a restrictive system of education and official examination by a central authority and to an elite Confucian society willing to tolerate, or unwilling or unable to challenge, that authority. Instead, already ancient medical knowledge in the *Huang Ti Nei Ching Su Wen* was altered and amended by learned scribes to become authoritative medical canon for a few elite practitioners. Emperors commissioned massive encyclopedic manuscripts of anecdotal herbal knowledge canvassed from their subjects. This is the knowledge that persisted up to, and was revived during, the twentieth century when the People's Republic of China adopted it as a cheap alternative to Western

---

[3] Veith, I., *Huang Ti Nei Ching Su Wen; The Yellow Emperor's Classic of Internal Medicine*, Baltimore, 1949.

medicine, and, to the dismay of many, it has widely proliferated today as Traditional Chinese Medicine. The perennial itinerant practitioners caring for the great mass of the population have enjoyed a separate but unregulated and virtually unrecorded existence.

{5} The earliest historical record of Indian medicine, which has much of empirical worth, can be dated only to *ca*. 100 BC. Nevertheless, traditional Indian medicine, Ayurveda, is thought to have originated during the Vedic age and is found in the *Atharva Veda* that some place as early as 2000 BC. But with the advent Hinduism, *ca*. 500 BC, it came under the hegemony of the Brahmin, or priest, caste, even medical training being within their purview. The medical texts were then infused with elements of Hinduism that changed their initially rational nature features to numinous. Concomitantly there was centralization of medical authority within practitioner guilds that were integrated into regional monarchical governments. Despite the insertion of elements of Hippocratic medicine as a consequence of Alexandrian and Islamic intrusions into the subcontinent, traditional Indian medicine would have changed little up to the present time were it not for assimilation of elements of modern Western medicine since the 18th century. The popularity of Ayurveda in part rests on its being a less expensive alternative to scientific medicine.

{6} Moving halfway around the globe, the practice of medicine is barely definable in the ancient Americas. There is virtually no written medical literature. Some idea of the medical environment can be derived from figurines and herbal lore, but, with no evidence of communication between professionals, the conclusion is that, if there were practitioners, they were local medical empiricists. In many pre-Columbian societies shamans were positioned to influence social direction, but no evidence of medical organization, professional or otherwise, has been identified in pre-Columbian art or other archeological finds.

{7} Finally, in the contested lands between Mesopotamia and Egypt there arose epochal creeds and ideas. But historical assessment of their nomadic tribes is limited because of disruptions among their societies and the disappearance of perishable textual materials. The Bible is the principal source of their histories, in part supported by archeological finds, in part at odds with them. Amid the flux of cultures and migratory tribes just to the east of the Mediterranean it is ancient Hebrew medicine that is best documented, and that can be credited to religious writings which began to accumulate in the 8th C BC. Notable features of Hebrew medicine were (1) intolerance of magical devices, and (2) a distinction between medical practitioners and priests. Although the nature of medical practice is uncertain, it probably had rational as well as empirical components. An unsettled tribal existence explains why a formal, and ultimately scientific, medical organization did not develop. Roman domination provided the colophon to indigenous medical practices. A profound inhibitory effect on medical progress has often been attributed to religions, and it is with this in mind that the Levant has been chosen to conclude this brief overview of primitive and ancient historical authoritarian societies and their effects on medical practice, for it was Hebrew prophets who first began to neutralize earthly authoritarianism using the morality of the individual as judged by an almighty God, thus opening a path to social equality. The profound consequences of this to medicine will be explained.

{8} In conclusion, a review of selected ancient civilizations suggests that several had evidence of a transient period in their earliest histories consistent with a rational medical practice. But within authoritarian society medicine did not benefit from the social advantages of a metropolis or the efficiency of centralized services, inevitably becoming, with the limited exception of Hebrew medicine, manipulated canon. None of the regions cited can claim precedence in originating a natural state of medical practice or of progress toward scientific medicine for none reached a steady state beyond that of the empirical. But the unheralded arrival of a new political system was soon to challenge, then surpass in greatness, all that had gone before.

{9}   The societal strata, or coordinates, of reasoning can be broadly summarized by ancient Greek terms: μονολογιζομένος (monologizomenos, or *that which is being reasoned by a solitary individual*), ἀνισολογιζομένος (anisologizomenos, or *that which is being reasoned by unequals*), and κοινολογιζομένος (koinologizomenos, or *that which is being reasoned in common council*). The first describes empiricism of the individual in primitive society, the second introduces the ruler or patron that characterizes authoritarian relationships, and the third describes a consequence of the democratic trend that first developed in ancient Hellas. Mycenaean Greece (1600-1100 BC), the Greek Dark Ages (1100-750 BC), and the early part of the Archaic Period (750-500 BC) provide little evidence for rational Greek medicine. But by the 5th C BC matters had dramatically changed. Many Greek city-states demonstrated broad acceptance of democratic governance. This preference demonstrated the principle of κοινονία (from "koinon," or *common council*)[4], and it was applied not just to government by the people, but also to political, trade, and craft associations. Simultaneously there emerged the availability of, and a public preference for, community practitioners of rational medicine, as corroborated by Thucydides' description of the plague of Athens.[5]

{10}   Preceding paragraphs have exposed authoritarian management of medicine as a guarantor of its survival but not its progress. In Greece the advance through monarchy, aristocracy, tyranny, and thence to democracy reflected political progress in Athens and other Hellenic city-states. Concurrently, medical practice progressed. In contrast, Sparta, which purposely chose to retain firm authoritarian, essentially communistic, governance, remained silent in medicine as in other things despite its proximity to Athens. It was at this time that the medical profession opened its ranks to those outside the traditional medical families. But it was the democratization of medical practice itself, the interaction of physician and patient rather than the admission of outsiders, that led to: (1) the recognition of the uniqueness of each patient, (2) the recognition of the complexity of diseases, and (3) acknowledgement of the patient's role in contributing to and directing his own medical care. This democratization of Hellenic medicine, often attributed to Hippocrates, represented the beginning of the true physician-patient relationship, the *natural state of medical practice*. In this κοινόν (koinon) of two it was not the physician's role that had changed; it was the patient's role, a revolutionary transformation. Engaged in common council against illness, the patient and physician could contribute equally to decision-making, the physician being the advocate for his patient and for no one else. It is argued that the honorable physician with such an obligation is far preferable to the legislated physician of an amoral State.

{11}   Because of the profound development in medical practice described above, Hippocrates has become the legendary icon for the modern physician. But the association of Hippocratic medicine with the modest Doric settlement on the eastern Mediterranean

---

[4] Koinon: an autonomous voluntary and democratic group sharing a common self-interest that meets in common council to freely exchange information and experience relevant to that self-interest and pertinent to all its members.

[5] My translation of the appropriate sections is found in vol. 2 of *The Natural State of Medical Practice*, p. 519.

island of Cos is unexpected, for neither geography nor demographics support the idea of a "medical school" on that small island. A more likely source for the origin of medical enlightenment was the ancient city of Miletos (romanized spelling of the Greek), located on the coast of Ionia about fifty miles from Cos, before it was laid waste by the Persians in 494 BC. But wherever its origin, Hippocratic medicine, which many consider the foundation of modern scientific medicine, is shown to be an indigenous Hellenic product, owing nothing whatsoever to prior or contemporary civilizations.

{12}   A lifetime in medicine affords limited opportunity for the tedious acquisition, by first-hand clinical experience, of new data or observations sufficient for publication. Thus, Hippocrates and Galen, as individuals, have received far too much credit for making medical discoveries. The lionization of these two early physicians is to a great extent attributable to the naivete or clinical incompetence of their medical successors, translators and biographers. It is obvious that complex clinical analyses from assembled observations of Hippocratic physicians were used to transcend the limitations of individual clinical experience. Within the collective experience of the Hippocratic physicians' association, or koinon, the correctness of so many medical analyses is shown to be proof that scientific revision, *i.e.*, confirmation of or improvement on preexisting knowledge, was made over time. The profession of medicine could now be defined as a science as well as an art and a profession.

{13, 14} Early Greek clinicians, who, like the early sophists, were peripatetic, understood that diseases of civilization were not god-inflicted, a prerequisite for rational medicine. With population growth and enlarging cities enabling physicians to cease their itinerant existence, the profession became more responsive to societal pressures but remained uninhibited by official entanglements. Therapeutic options were limited, and the pharmacopoeia was small, the latter reflecting a critical assessment of its components by Hippocratic physicians rather than the massive lists of supposed medicaments posed in other civilizations. Medicine was a profession requiring hard work to obtain a livelihood, and the Hippocratic practitioner engaged in both medical and surgical treatments. Thus, by the 4th C BC medicine was an unattractive livelihood for the upper classes, although there was familiarity with its theories by intellectuals of the day.

{15}   With regard to societal pressures and the Hippocratic Oath, there are profound limits on the assistance that a person can expect from a stranger unless society establishes, by custom or by laws, a form of compensation for the stranger. *Compassion*, as a modern "virtue" and viewed as commanding some vague form of intrinsic emotional compensation and one traditionally identified with medicine, holds no special place in that profession, and can at times be counterproductive, a problem identified by the Hippocratics. More important by far is humaneness, a "kinship of all sentient life expressed through kindness and mercy." This was a component of many ancient philosophical doctrines, but it expressed the thinking of but a few individual philosophers who, living in authoritarian societies, devised those doctrines and wished to inculcate humaneness into their followers. In contrast, Greek humaneness became a component of daily life concurrently with individual liberty. Although no discoverer of this virtue, the Greeks, as a society, elevated humaneness from philosophy to action. The reason, of course, is that virtue is impossible in the absence of freedom of choice. It was, therefore, the Greeks that injected humaneness into medicine. The Hippocratic Oath was not intended to mold a physician into the perfect man; it was a humane working document outlining the physician's obligations, and its enforcement was based on trust.

{16}   But concurrently with the decline of Greek city-state democracies, a process that began in the 4th C BC, Greek medicine became less attractive as a profession over the next two centuries, and fewer practitioners were identified with the island of Cos and Hippocrates. Concurrently, in ascendant Rome scientific medicine never became an established vocation. As Rome embraced the Mediterranean, its medicine was for the most part provided by alternative (non-Hippocratic) practitioners, often Greek, a process well-advanced as the Common Era opened and virtually complete shortly thereafter. It was against these incompetents that Galen (2nd C AD) railed.

{17} Possible reasons for the loss of Hippocratic medicine are presented, but only one seems adequate to the task. Early in the 1st C BC Roman guilds (collegia) became increasingly regulated by the State that frowned on plebeian organizations in general and Greek organizations in particular. Thus, in addition to a diminishing number of Hippocratic physicians concurrent with a declining and destabilized Greece, the proximate cause of the loss of scientific medicine was the medical profession's inability to sustain, within the Roman world, the medical koinon, or venue of common council, as a source for medical excellence. The medical koinon would have provided a focus for public esteem and, thereby, recruitment. In its absence medical attrition was quantitative rather than qualitative, but it was complete. After the Caesars and their successors were replaced by a theocratic bureaucracy nothing filled the void produced by the disappearance of the Hippocratic clinician as the Dark Ages approached.

{18, 19} Absent the rediscovery of classic authors there is little to recommend the European Dark Ages (400-1000 AD) and High Medieval period (1000-1300 AD), at least in the field of medicine. This is vividly supported by the dearth of medical discovery and the short life expectancy. Hippocratic medical practice in the Eastern Roman Empire was never established, and with the fall of the Western Roman Empire and the onset of the Dark Ages in Europe medicine became the work of the layman. Medicine as a profession had become extinct. Much Hippocratic learning was preserved by 6th C Nestorians in Gondeshapour (Jondi-Shapur), passing in subsequent centuries into Persian and Islamic hands and then slowly reentering Europe by the 11th C. Humanists then reopened the books of ancient scholarship, but this would have led to little had not medieval Europe retraced the political steps of ancient Hellas, passing sequentially through feudalism, aristocracy, and then tyranny in the guise of the Italian Renaissance. Thus, with a growing population and the creation of independent European city-states, medical practitioners organized through guilds and university faculties. But, instilling the words rather than the concepts of Hippocratic medicine, they produced, even through the 17th C, only the facade of a profession.

{20, 21} There did occur, however, a transient period with a burst of individualism in the Renaissance as select individuals offered a glimpse of the potential for genius that lay concealed for 1500 years. Often independent of ideas handed down from ancient physicians and natural philosophers, a few individuals were able to initiate studies of their own design. But consistent with the social pattern of the age, fine arts, architecture, music, and science were supported by the patron, a wealthy or prominent individual who afforded both protection and support for his favorites, expecting in most cases some public acknowledgement and secondary gain from his benevolence. Nevertheless, although the patron's support was a vital force in Renaissance discovery, it is shown that Renaissance medical discovery amounted to nothing of consequence for future ages.

{22} The vast abyss that was the medicine of the Dark Ages was finally traversed. Nevertheless, the impotence of medical progress persisted. It would remain to the resurgence of individualism, as reflected in the 16th C Reformation and the 17th C appreciation of natural law and natural rights, to bring forth the 18th C miracle of progress that has continued to this day.

When Martin Luther posted his ninety-five theses on the door of All Saints' Church in 1517 a massive stumbling block to progress was removed. Within three years his message, profoundly aided by the recent invention of the printing press, engaged much of Europe in a reordering of religious institutions. And the power behind this change was recognition of the individual's personal association with God. No longer would the common man and woman be constrained adherents of a pan-European doctrinal kinship distributed among fiefdoms. The importance of the individual was not a new idea in the West. Thomas Aquinas (1225-1274) had viewed each person as having free will. But subsequent to the Reformation and concurrent with the emergence in Europe of elements of democracy as manifested in 17th and 18th century parliaments a *bona fide* medical practice appeared, just as it had 2300 years earlier in ancient Greece. Arising from the feudalism of the Dark Ages and Medieval Period, the increasingly liberated common citizenry now had opportunities for displaying their genius, including medical practice.

{23}   Western Europe and Great Britain were the sites for this reincarnation of the Hippocratic koinon of Cos. Autonomous professional organizations and medical journals improved the work of the medical profession. Discoveries would now be vetted by the new koinons, and physicians began to successfully compete with the medicine-men of their day. It was the unencumbered physician and his organizations, not the Renaissance, that would bring about a second approximation to the *natural state of medical practice*. Herein is found support for the assertion that modern medicine would have progressed to its present point even without Hippocrates or the Renaissance. It is shown that in each of three eras (Greco-Roman, Renaissance, and Modern) equivalent discoveries were not only made, but were made independent of any prior discoveries and without sophisticated technology. A logical corollary is that many seminal discoveries and inventions of the 18th and 19th centuries could just as well have been made prior to the Common Era had freedom for the individual and for group associations (the koinons) prevailed in the Greco-Roman world.

{24}   The role of medical journals in the history of medicine has received inadequate attention, for it is the medical journal, as the mouthpiece of the medical koinon, that brought back the natural state of medical practice. Whereas the Renaissance inventor and his patron relied on distribution of a relatively small number of books, usually written in Latin, to a relatively small number of friends, associates, and prominent persons, the democratic and vernacular medical journal was available to professionals in all reaches of society, the phenomenal result being that koinons now had an international range and were thereby internationally productive to the benefit of all mankind.

{25}   But progress is not inevitable and the authoritarian is again on the march, this time on a global scale. Today's phenomenal technology of medicine is a product of capitalism and will thrive only within a capitalistic system, and *the natural state of medical practice*, which is the stimulus for that technology, is a product of a free society. Today the practitioner finds himself increasingly regulated, and it is ironic that the regulation stems from the profession's increasingly porous boundaries. Medicine's immigrants are becoming medicine's masters. The Hippocratic Oath is increasingly irrelevant, the work of the profession is ever more performed by those with inferior training, the professional organization is diluted by nonphysicians, medical practice is managed by nonphysicians, medical care is distributed by nonphysicians, and, with the prize of medicine ever more fame and fortune, the attractions of a career in medicine are those of a business or a competition rather than a profession. The root of the problem lies not with those outside the profession who see advantage in a medical alliance. It lies, instead, with the profession that seeks them out. The koinon that guided the practice of medicine from superstition to science must redefine its limits and, reversing a sixty-year trend in America, cease being bigger and start getting better.

PART II
Prehistoric Analysis

{26}   But what initiated valid medical practices in the first place, specifically those of Mesopotamia, Egypt, China, India, and Greece? Given the present subject, its huge volume and its vast unknowns, the opening chapter for Part II offers such justification for its examination and interpretation of prehistoric civilizations and their medical progress as is seemly for a clinical physician with an eye to the dearth of effective medical care over the ages. But to better assess prehistoric primary civilizations and proto-civilizations it is first necessary to return to, and focus on, the formative years of those historic civilizations for which evidence of medical progress, transient as it was, still exists. If common characteristics associated with their success can be identified, those same characteristics can then be sought in prehistoric civilizations.

{27}   The history of Miletos from its founding until its razing by the Persians in 494 BC is briefly reviewed with a focus on its early governance and commercial enterprise. Miletos, arising *de novo* in the 11th C BC is selected as a paradigm population for an attempt at understanding the origin of the medical successes of Hippocratic Greece, for the home island of Hippocrates, Cos, can be excluded as the origin of Hippocratic medicine. Milesian medical practitioners of the 6th C BC are assumed to have been the source of at least some of the earlier clinical observations found in the Hippocratic Corpus, although it would be reasonable to assign a similar course of political, commercial, and medical practice developments to other city-states in ancient Ionia and the Dodecanese Islands. Selected metrics and observations, including population size and density, physical area, area of hegemony, governance, monuments, and life expectancy, are then summarized, against which sixteen other urbanized or proto-urbanized primary civilizations will be compared.

{28}   Sumer is the first of four great primary civilizations to be compared to Miletos. The prehistory of Sumer and the founding and rise of its largest city-state, Uruk, are presented, and the early agricultural and commercial prosperity of that city before conquest by Akkadians (2350 BC) is proposed as the social milieu in which a network of medical practitioners acquired the ancient wisdom of clinical medicine that would find its way into later Babylonian medical writings. Extant writings and legend suggest that the independent *azu* ("physician") was recognized as a commendable member of society probably as early as 3200 BC (during the Late Uruk Period), although a mature cuneiform probably was unavailable to record his observations until *ca.* 2800 BC. Scholarly literature has a number of fine articles revealing the clinical acuity of presumably Sumerian clinicians, and I review one exceptional example in detail. The rise of an autonomous city-state at a time of (1) weakening of egalitarian kinship ties, (2) commercial prosperity, and (3) prior to authoritarian centralization of political power is proposed as containing the window of opportunity for autonomous specialization, and this would include the formation of a medical koinon, or medical network capable of initiating medical progress.

{29}   In Egypt the original compositions that would be transcribed *ca.* 1550 BC and subsequently known as the Ebers and Smith medical papyri can be traced to the Proto-Dynastic (3300-3085 BC) or Early Dynastic periods of Egyptian history, at least for *Papyrus Ebers*. In addition to linguistic evidence, reasons for this claim are presented, the principal one being the status of society adjacent to the unification of Egypt under the Pharaohs (3085 BC), a period noted for flourishing commercial manufacture, population growth, and prosperity. As the largest urban area along the Nile prior to unification, the city-state of Hierakonpolis is selected as the most likely site for the acquisition and collation of medical wisdom that is present in the two famous medical papyri. The dissimilarity between Sumerian cuneiform and Egyptian hieroglyphic and hieratic clinical descriptions does not support the notion that Egyptian medicine was an importation from the Mesopotamian civilization.

{30}   Recent archeology has revealed the remarkable remnants of an Indus River Valley civilization that may parallel in scope the Mesopotamian civilization. In contrast to Uruk, the minimal evidence of fortifications and social stratification provide traditional support for an egalitarian social organization in the region for much of its history. The prospering Indus River Valley civilization had access to the Arabian Sea, to central Asia, east through the sub-Himalayan belt across the Indian subcontinent, and to the tropical south. New findings indicate the local culture, rather than an Indo-Aryan immigration, was the likely source of at least a portion of the Vedas that have guided Indian culture ever since. The principal relevance to medicine has been the *Atharva Veda*, the foundation of Ayurvedic medicine. The *Charaka Samhita* and the *Sushruta Samhita*, roughly 2,000 years old, are the classic expressions of Ayurvedic medicine, and they contain a wealth of clinical material unfortunately rewritten over the ages to support a theocratic elite class, the Brahman. But the original objective observations in the two works probably derive from the Vedic age when the Indus River Valley civilization was commercially flourishing (2600-2000 BC), suggesting the presence during that period of a network of medical practitioners that had evolved in its early cities. That such medical acumen was of rural acquisition following the decline of that civilization is untenable.

{31}   Again looking eastward, legend holds that it was in the time of the Yellow Emperor (*ca.* 2500 BC) that the Chinese medical classic, the *Huang Ti Nei Ching Su Wen*, a dialogue between the Yellow Emperor and his ministers, was composed. Although modern documentation places its composition *ca.* 150 BC, its contents were considered already ancient at that time. Confucius (6th C BC) was able to identify a "good physician" from a "good wizard," suggesting rational medicine had evolved in earlier centuries. The traditional location of the Yellow Emperor is northeastern China. An example of the contemporary Longshan culture city-state in that region is Liangchengzhen, a prominent coastal commercial center and one postulated by archeologists, in part from the nature of its ceramics, to be relatively free from centralized authoritarian control. Although no medical presence has so far been uncovered from archeological sites, it is proposed that the medical observations in the *Huang Ti Nei Ching Su Wen* were first made in such an urban environment. Over the centuries substantial new content was amended and emended. But underneath the "new age" additions and the heavy editing in the 8th C AD by Wang Bing, a nonphysician, the practical, and sometimes acute, observations made by those ancient practitioners can be detected. These, the true authors of the authentic portions of the *Huang Ti Nei Ching Su Wen*, will remain unknown, but we can opine about the social world in which they worked.

{32}   In reviewing the preceding four famed civilizations a distinction must be made between so-called "great" civilizations and primary civilizations, the former being sequences of regional civilizations that do not progress over time but their apparent longevity and wealth, achieved by conquest and exploitation, is viewed as a manifestation of "greatness." A primary civilization, however, arises *de novo*, is independent of any pre-existing civilization, and has the freedom to lay the groundwork for subsequent prosperity before authoritarian centralization of political power occurs. Each of the four "great civilizations" began as a primary civilization. The four primary civilizations of the "great" civilizations, all of which had city-states, are compared to the ancient Greek city-state of Miletos with regard to size of the local population, the regional population, population density, city area, time to prosperity, life expectancy, duration of greatest flourishing, and governance, *inter alia*. The term "heterarchy" is introduced.[6] This is followed by a discussion of cities and urbanization.

{33}   Then, after defining a "lesser" civilization, there is an explanation for the selection of twelve prehistoric civilizations and proto-civilizations for analysis, including a discussion of the significance of alluvial environments, geography, reasons for non-selection, and issues related to identifying form of governance. A precis of each of the twelve lesser civilizations is then given, along with a list of the same metrics and other characteristics that were applied to the five historical civilizations. This is followed by a summary of those characteristics relevant to present purpose.

{34}   With data now in hand, limited and circumstantial as it is, discussion focuses on lifestyle decisions and urbanization. Following the Late Neolithic, it took several thousands of years before personal preferences led to agricultural settlements and village life. Commercialization then led to urbanization. But with one possible exception a most remarkable finding is that in none of the twelve prehistoric civilizations/proto-civilizations was there evidence of formalized medical care or medical care of any kind. This was so despite the long duration and large size of some of their well-defined population centers, *e.g.*, Catalhoyuk (8th millennium BC Anatolia, population 8,000-10.000, duration >1,000 years), Djenne-djenno (1st millennium AD sub-Saharan Africa, population 50,000, duration 600 years), Cucuteni-Trypillia (4th millennium BC eastern Europe, centers with populations of 10,000-30,000, duration 1,000 years). This is compared to the two or three centuries over which ancient Greece and the modern West moved from simple medical empiricism to scientific understanding. Then are discussed the Australian aborigines who, with their strong kinship ties, have for perhaps 50,000 years failed to develop either medical practitioners or a single town.

A separate issue is life expectancy, and of those seventeen civilizations for which there are data, the average life expectancy, based on archeologically estimated age at death, is little more than thirty years for the common man and woman, and children usually did not know their grandparents, a sad commentary on social organizations of the human species in the past but a spectacular comment on the freedom of Western nations where life expectancy now approximates eighty years and great-great- grandparents are not rare.

A statistical assessment of data from the seventeen civilizations in Part II receives a more extensive analysis in the unabridged publication of this work, but from its most significant conclusions, (1) statistically the most likely explanation for the failure to initiate progress in ancient primary civilizations is the egalitarian kinship system, and (2) a tentative list of demographic requirements for initiation of a nascent medical profession in a primary civilization includes:

---

[6] Heterarchy: A multifocal system of management in a social system in which there is no permanent head.

1. A collegial network of at least several medical practitioners
2. Two or three centuries of social stability
3. Prosperity, as evidenced by trade and specialization, sufficient to support medical practitioners working for profit
4. A localized population in the tens of thousands, perhaps as low as 10,000

But for this overview social factors will now receive our attention.

{35}   Egalitarianism is closely examined because its effects are greatest in that segment of ancient populations from which medical practitioners arose, the unprivileged, or commoner class. Definitions of egalitarianism are discussed, with social egalitarianism as a practical answer to social organization in early and primitive societies. With permanent settlements, specific archeological characteristics help scholars identify the more egalitarian communities. As for the mechanism by which an egalitarian social organization existed in the first place, Maslow's system of motivational hierarchy is discussed. The primal levels of the hierarchy, survival and safety, are pressing personal motivations and are considered irrelevant to egalitarianism. But now the "need to belong" motivation comes into play as each member attempts to adapt to, or modify the behavior of, others to accommodate his or her own behavioral preferences. At some point the more forcefully impelled or popularly held opinion restricts opposing ones. Thus, a seemingly democratic result in an egalitarian society can shut down all alternatives. Primacy of the band or tribe over the individual also demands redistribution, another inhibitor of progress. But it is concluded that the evil aspects of egalitarianism decrease as trade promotes urbanization, prosperity, and population growth. It does this because urbanization, being solely a consequence of commercial ventures, weakens kinship allegiances and provides a window of opportunity for individuals and families to break free.

{36}   To break free from the kinship means that individuals now can respond to their own needs rather than those of their leader or their society. It also provides a more discernable opportunity for implementation of natural law. Following a definition of natural law that includes its applicability to all mankind, it is axiomatic that it must apply equally to both early and modern man, including ancient hunter-gatherers. As far as it is a "law," it exists to assist social man, and to do this it protects the individual. Because of the varying definitions of natural law, the term as used here is equated with the *moral sense* as described by Dr. James Q. Wilson.[7] Evidence supporting the existence and general applicability of natural law in historical and modern societies is reviewed. Its relevance to early human societies and the consequences of actions in accordance with, or inconsistent with, natural law as they affect the development of primitive society are then discussed. The conclusion is that coercive egalitarianism and egalitarian kinships include within their strategies infringements on individual freedom inconsistent with natural law and are therefore immoral. It is argued that they inhibit proper societal evolution and the realization of progress. Natural law functions, through the undirected effort of individuals, to assist communal good, but it is easily displaced by passion, rhetorical persuasion and threats. Sadly, as a consequence, the felonies of a few have, over thousands of years, devolved great misery upon the many.

{37}   The role of writing in promoting progress is reviewed and it is concluded that inscribed symbols first develop as a tool for commercial operation, but proper writing is

---

[7] Wilson, J. Q., *The Moral Sense*, New York, 1993.

a sign of progress rather than a cause of progress. In this sense it can be equated with a medical practice as an early marker of progress. Once matured, the usefulness of the tool is remarkable to the point that it becomes, unexpectedly, an intellectual end in itself, an example of spontaneous order, an unintended good. In contrast to writing, it is the formation of small autonomous groups promoting self-interest that, although developing in parallel with writing, are the true initiators of progress. Both writing and the small autonomous group were conceived by breaking egalitarian kinship bonds as commerce first appeared in settled societies. The optimal small autonomous group is the koinon, and its features, discussed early in this work, are repeated. It is proposed that independent self-interest groups are more likely in a heterarchical society because such a society permits individuals to forego previous allegiances and thereby be free to pursue specialized self-betterments that evolve as part of what social scientists call a "settlement hierarchy."[8]

{38}   Concluding Part II, after a definition of historicism and a review of its criticisms, it is argued that historicism may justifiably identify some basic threats to human progress and as an aspect of social science should not be discarded. It is further argued that historicism has yet to be fairly tested, for history has never recorded a "satisfactory" civilization; duration is surely not a guide. The negative social consequences of political authoritarianism on the maturation of progress (Part 1), and of egalitarianism on the initiation of progress (Part II), have been identified in this work. The importance of small groups to progress is discussed and the profound distinction between democracy and individualism is noted. Progress which emerged from release of the unprivileged, or commoner, citizenry was not the consequence of democracy. It was the consequence of freedom that permitted the voluntary autonomous group, fed and led by self-betterment, to discover and invent. That group, essential to specialization, is the koinon, and it finds its place at the pinnacle of a proposed new theory, the "Isagorial Theory of Human Progress."[9] Democracy is nonetheless useful, for it is the only form of governance that can accommodate the existence of koinons, meaning that it is the only form of governance that up to a point can resist the temptation to interfere with self-interest group activity. It is the not-so-subtle threat of today that such support can be withdrawn.

EPILOGUE

In recounting the history and prehistory of medical practice a pattern has fallen into place that was unintended at this work's inception, namely an insight into the social circumstances surrounding the evolution of medical practice. As demonstrated in the three volumes of *The Natural State of Medical Practice*, medical progress, used now as a surrogate for both pragmatic and intellectual progress, has always been prepared to emerge from the shadow of existential threats that can be acute, poignant, and demanding.

---

[8] Settlement hierarchy: the mechanism proposed as the natural way intergroup adjustments take place as an enlarging population center that has had no prior experience with a leadership hierarchy becomes more complex and must deal with new goods and services needed by the evolving society.
[9] *Isagorial Theory of Human Progress*: A theory ascribing all apolitical advances for the betterment of mankind to autonomous associations pursuing self-betterment in which each member has equal opportunity to speak freely and share ideas about the group's common interest without fear of retribution. Axiomatically it excludes "betterments" that have been stolen, copied, derived by exploitation, or used for subjugation of others.

The window of opportunity for that emergence, however, is small and vulnerable. Had it been otherwise, much advanced knowledge of a modern nature might have been available in what we now call prehistory. Indeed, the prehistoric human experience might have been significantly shorter had the escape from egalitarianism by our ancient forbears occurred sooner. Based on data from the Population Reference Bureau it can be estimated that 100 billion humans died between 50,000 BC and the 18th C AD, at which time the natural state of medical practice was reinstituted in the West and modern medicine and its scientific ramifications proceeded to mollify or prevent many of the miseries of humankind, dramatically improving what is bureaucratically termed QALY (Quality-Adjusted Life-Year), and doing so on a global scale.[10] It is a fair deduction, given the evidence in *The Natural State of Medical Practice*, that a significant proportion of those dying before the age of modern medicine would have had access to rational medical care had the escape from egalitarianism been successful thousands of years earlier. Absurd? Remember that rational/scientific medicine is, at its origin, simple, cheap, easy, convenient, and requires no technology, and everyone wishes it success.

Nevertheless, with the remarkable progress that has been made in the past three centuries, perhaps mankind has finally, and permanently, ridded itself of a self-imposed serfdom that has led to entrapment of the mass of humanity and has shuffled off all past civilizations to their demise. But in doing so it has left historians with only the history of authoritarian machinations and the monuments recording the tragedies of human folly rather than the story of the common man and woman from which to untangle the story of mankind. Thus, the question to be posed is not "what happened in our past." It is, instead, what did not happen. Although what did not happen will never be known, why matters happened as they did is now known. The root problem, having heretofore been overlooked, is demonstrated in the present work: authoritarianism in its many nefarious forms, one being social egalitarianism.

It is proposed that the recent efforts of the West, successful so far, and in retrospect the few and temporary successes of ancient times, can be attributed solely to liberty, but not of just liberty of the individual. More importantly for human progress, it is liberty of the autonomous group with focused self-betterment. The reason is simple: two heads are better than one.

The desire for and appreciation of liberty is inherent in every human heart, a component of the individual conscience traceable to natural law, that subtle human attribute that is neither genetic nor learned but has been available to all mankind since the first man and woman. Always, in the past, have authoritarian policies or doctrines pushed the good genie of our conscience back into the bottle as the authoritarian conscience ascended and asserted its own definition of right and wrong. In our age, however, a marvelous expansion of both progress and of an appreciation of liberty in promoting the welfare of all mankind can be dated to the commencement of the Reformation.[11] Indeed,

---

[10] See: Weinstein, M. C., Torrance, G., McGuire, A., *QALYs: The Basics*, in *Value in Health*, 12:S5-S9, 2009.

[11] Although one must wonder what the consequences of the early 19th C "invention" of socialism would have been had it been more successful in shaping social policies in the West prior to the work of Pasteur, Maxwell, Curie, Roentgen, Edison, and Einstein, among many others. It is probable, perhaps even certain, that many of the great discoveries and inventions that have produced our brave new world would never have transpired if egalitarian policies had full play in the early 19th C. The idea that somehow those discoveries and inventions were inevitable is a catastrophic misinterpretation of history. In their absence we might still have been living in Dickensian times.

it may be stated that *the natural state of medical practice*, as defined and historically interpreted herein, has contributed to unprecedented healthful longevity because of beneficent consequences from adherence to natural law.[12] Let us, then, reconsider our attribution of today's manifold successes to great empires, great cities, and great men, to ethnic forbears, and to central planning. It is nothing like that; they are but the headline-catching flotsam on the far more interesting sea of humanity. Rejoice in the accomplishments of genius, but forget not that genius has abounded in every age and in every people as a well-kept secret, and that every person, in the appropriate place and at the appropriate time, can be considered a genius at something. Indeed, the unique genius of *Homo sapiens* lies in its variations that are expressed best in the ability of that species to recognize the benefits of peaceful group deliberation by free individuals for their varied ideas with a goal of self-interest focusing on the problem at hand. Unfortunately, it has been the rule of the jungle or the mob, *i.e.*, to take from or to control others, that has consistently delayed the establishment, or speeded the demise, of that principle of genius.

Briefly put, the broad-based success we enjoy in the West today, especially in healthful longevity, has been acquired in little more than two or three centuries. The road map for that success has been identified: in history and prehistory the course of *the natural state of medical practice* coincides with the course of liberty of the individual. That liberty allows expression of the innate genius of our species as magnified through various human agencies. But present success is sporadic and human history suggests it is not permanent, for the unceasing authoritarian quest for control over, and uniformity of, every human endeavor using all necessary means of coercion remains today an increasingly threatening presence at home and globally. As we look about us today and witness the massive influx of foreign populations into Western democracies, an influx variously attributed to seeking asylum, fleeing poverty, and evading humanitarian disasters, what we are seeing is nothing more than an escape from egalitarianism and its consequences, the principal difference today being both the magnitude of the problem and the frantic efforts being made by egalitarian's emigrant who now knows, by virtue of modern communication, that he or she need not chance survival alone in the jungle or on the savannah when they leave their kinship or comradeship, but that in that country just across the border there is a better life, liberty, and the possibility of happiness. More than just medical practice is in the balance.

But there is an even greater revelation here. The Reformation initiated two unanticipated parallel but complementary events: (1) it set the West on the path toward technical progress as mankind was gradually able to implement its collective genius, and (2) by freeing up mankind's ability to freely consult its collective conscience, it directed that path toward a secular Eden, a free and prosperous society. Unfortunately, the march of events in modern times indicates that path to be less and less likely to be travelled for long.

[12] The cause of the "healthful longevity" is due, of course, not just to medical diagnosis and treatment, but also to biological knowledge and supportive sciences upon which rest disease prevention, sanitation, epidemiology, nutrition, food supply, workplace safety, and veterinary services, among many others. The success of medicine is but a marker for the status of progress on many fronts within a population.

EXCURSUS 2

This excursus, a summary of the political implications of *The Natural State of Medical Practice*, is an "opening salvo" for much that follows. It identifies the role of descriptive science, or "inductive" reasoning, in the work's conclusions, the relevance of human freedom to natural law, and, supported by statistical proof, the essential role of the unprivileged but free "common man and woman" to human progress as gauged by life expectancy. The conclusion targets modern-day threats to that progress.

INDUCTIVE PROOF OF THE ESSENTIAL ROLE OF LIBERTY AND LIMITED GOVERNMENT IN HUMAN PROGRESS

Beyond mere economic efficiency, contemporary argument favoring limited government is based on evidence of government dysfunction (negative evidence) and on societal improvements that follow governmental deregulation (positive evidence). The persuasiveness of this argument is bolstered by appeal to tenets of theoretical political philosophies that argue individual liberty is an inherent right or gift of God, an end also consistent with limited government. The latter appeals represent *deductive* reasoning as derived from philosophical or religious principles or dogma, often supported by reference to the contentious subject of natural law.[1] There has, however, been presented no justification for limited governance of a society solely using *inductive* reasoning, *i.e.*, based on historical facts that provide a scientific proof of the beneficial effect of limited governance. The three-volume work, *The Natural State of Medical Practice*, provides such a proof.

Some years ago while on the staff of a large municipal hospital in New York City I began to study the history of earlier medical practices with the intention of finding clues that could improve unsatisfactory aspects of modern medical care in the United States. Unexpectedly, I discovered that the deleterious issues throughout the history of medicine were not of medical origin, instead being attributable to social issues, primarily stemming from authoritarian governance. In the "great civilizations" of Mesopotamia, Egypt, India, and China, authoritarian governments or institutions commandeered

---

[1] For example, Objectivists view what is generally considered "natural rights" as "objective rights," the latter term being a matter of definition and an analytical approach of a philosophy. But the argument and proof posed in this excursus is not philosophical. It is, instead, rational in that it is derived by induction from observed events. As a piece of induction, it can then be considered for a place within a theory from which issues might then be deduced. Natural rights/natural law, whether God-given or derived from the rational mind of man, might be considered such a theory. The present excursus provides positive support for the theory. For Objectivism, however, it appears to be irrelevant to any validation of philosophical theory, for it can be argued that Objectivism requires no such validation. If one concludes, therefore, that the argument of the excursus is convincing, it strengthens the case for natural rights/natural law but not for Objectivism. In the former it is a formal supportive proof to be further studied; for the latter it is but to be expected, and if it does not provide such proof the philosophical strength of Objectivism is unimpaired. As a "positivist" approach by proponents of natural rights/natural law one might consider the former more appealing in that objectivity is its nature. This suggests a curious anomaly in Objectivism.

medical practices that had evolved during their early primary civilizations (*de novo* civilizations not shaped by dependence on or control by other more complex societies) to serve their own purposes. There were but two exceptions to this *political authoritarianism* in the historical record: Hippocratic medicine in ancient Greece (transient) and modern Western medicine (still operative.)

I then sought even earlier medical practices. With the reasonable conjecture that modern humans assumed their place on this planet perhaps 50,000 years ago, I looked at medical practices in prehistory, assuming there was no logical reason to think that prehistoric *Homo sapiens* was less intelligent than are we. In brief, reviewing scholarly reports covering twelve primary urban or proto-urban civilizations ranging from 8th millennium BC to 1300 AD I found no evidence of formal medical practice, even though three of the twelve prehistoric civilizations each endured for more than a thousand years. Simple statistical analyses applied to the necessarily limited and sometimes circumstantial data on hand supported the conclusion that initiation of formal medical practices was profoundly inhibited by a different expression of authoritarianism, the *social egalitarianism* of the kinship.[2] Australian aborigines, having an isolated existence for perhaps 50,000 years without formal medical practices and without forming a single town, can be viewed as contemporary evidence for this claim. Thus, the common denominator opposing medical progress has always been authoritarianism in either its political or egalitarian guise.

Over all eras, it was demonstrated that an effective collegial medical practice (termed the *natural state of medical practice*) has arisen solely from efforts of the common citizenry. On their liberation, periods of documentable medical progress occurred *briefly* during early urbanization (the "settlement hierarchy" phase) of the primary city-states of Mesopotamia, Egypt, India and China prior to centralization of power, *substantially* during the early democracies of Classical Greece, and *definitively* in late 18th C Western civilization during its march to democracy that began when the Reformation curtailed a pan-European doctrinal kinship that had existed for more than a thousand years. As corollaries, it was demonstrated (1) that Hippocratic medicine has been irrelevant to modern medical progress, (2) that the Renaissance with its patronage by tyrants has been of no consequence to medical progress, and (2) that the recent phenomenal lengthening of life expectancy around the globe is solely the result of Western scientific medicine and method as it has been stealthily intercalated into local and traditional health practices.

Thus, it has been inductively proven that medical progress is associated with and attributable to one thing, and one thing only: freedom of the common man and woman.[3] Furthermore, this proof is supported indirectly in that the absence of liberty is associated with only occasional medical observations or empirical remedies that might temporarily help a circumscribed population but would not be propagated or improved, regardless of how long a society endures.

Remarkably, from the course of medical discovery in early Classical Greece and in the 18th C West, the rise of efficient scientific discovery from ignorance and simple empiricism is shown to require, under appropriate circumstances, only two or three

---

[2] The details of this analysis are to be found in vol. 3 of *The Natural State of Medical Practice*, p. 313*f.*

[3] It is understood that the strength of inductive reasoning relies on the confirmation of earlier findings. That is the reason for presenting a website, **contratyrannos.com**, to the general public: the seeking of arguments *pro* and *con*.

centuries. Furthermore, the mechanism for discovery of basic truths of scientific medicine practice is easy, cheap, simple, and convenient: the medical history and physical examination. It is, instead, external interference with collegial collection, dissemination, integration and coordination of clinical knowledge that has always been the problem.

But there is more. Because pain and suffering are equally felt in all societies and at all levels of a society, they should provoke a similar response in all societies and lead to a nascent discipline of medicine as people work together to seek solutions to problems at hand. This is so basic that a failure to do so suggests a systemic inability to progress in any discipline, the term "progress" being defined as awareness of the improvability of the communal status. This incompetence, of course, can be masked in societies/civilizations that survive and thrive by conquest, theft and deceit. It is concluded that medical practice is a surrogate for intellectual and technical progress in general. If this is the case, the arguments presented in this series of monographs can also be considered inductive proof for the existence of natural law in addition to being its consequence. When natural law, which I argue is an inviolable statement on individual liberty, is disobeyed by the politically powerful, progress is not possible.

But how can the common citizenry, the unprivileged, be the source of progress? *The Natural State of Medical Practice* provides abundant examples showing genius, defined as exceptional natural ability, is neither rare nor discriminative; it is profusely spread over all humankind. Left alone, the common man and woman will devise, discover, and invent, a process vastly accelerated if they are not inhibited from forming autonomous collaborative groups to exploit a common self-interest. Everyone bears the potential for genius, a unique biological variable found only in *Homo sapiens* and one that may not be apparent unless the requisite opportunity appears. Alternative theories of progress, whether attributed to "great men," "great empires," "great cities" or ethnic forebears, are either wrong or are the consequence of, rather than cause of, progress. Had humankind earlier broken through the opaque ceiling of authoritarianism, our ancestors would, for generations or even millennia, have had some effective alleviation of suffering from disease, difficult childbirth and injury. The full extent of this authoritarian tragedy is unfathomable.

The question arises as to present-day significance of the proof just reviewed. Many of today's problems arise from centralization of political power that subsumes personal liberty and responsibility. The medical profession is itself partly responsible for its own problems in that it has, over the last seventy-five years, invited that intrusion. Even the Hippocratic Oath, a personal promise of the physician to the individual patient, is being reinterpreted to fit authoritarian convenience. The authoritarian is always on the march, this time on a global scale, and the threat to common men and women around the world is great. The magnitude of that threat over the ages is exposed in *The Natural State of Medical Practice*.

EXCURSUS 3

By interpreting natural law as a statement on the inviolability of human liberty, identification of infractions of natural law become less subjective. In this excursus a proof is offered that identifies natural law as purposeful and beneficial because both increased life expectancy and an effective collegial medical association are shown to be products of human liberty. It is also confirmed that natural law is an attribute of all mankind and unrelated to race, ethnicity, unique characteristics, or social class. It concludes with the observation that natural law as a protection of natural rights in secular governance in the West, despite its limited extent and whether intended or not, has spread a beneficence of natural law globally. The tragic consequences should it be lost are predicted.

ISAGORIAL THEORY OF HUMAN PROGRESS AS A PROOF OF NATURAL LAW AND ITS BENEFICENCE

Introduction

The foundation of natural law assumes there is free will and that there lies within every individual a moral sense that helps us distinguish between good and evil when we make our choices. Its realm of importance, therefore, includes choices pertinent to our personal lives and, through participation, in political choices. The tendency to congruence of natural law with English common law has been considered a reflection of the good effect of conscience in justifying the development of legal precedent over many centuries.

Attempts have been made to define what is good or evil under natural law and thereby to fashion laws sympathetic to that concept. But just what is considered good or evil is not always clear-cut, and this has led to disputation about the merits of natural law, in part because it has been viewed by some as a list of things not to do, and proposed lists are not consistent.[1] There is, however, a common thread that runs through all proposals: do not trespass on the rights of others, including their "right" to life (do not murder) and property (do not steal/covet). Using this as a nonspecific interpretation of natural law, it is reasonable to consider it not as a list of things not to do but as *a statement on the inviolability of individual liberty*. Assessment of good or evil under natural law, which some define as the law of reason, thereby becomes less a matter of opinion if a question can be framed in terms of infringement of individual liberty. Legal implications and issues then become more like matters of boundary rather than definition.

From the preceding it can also be argued that natural law is but a guide for protection of the individual. To do this it delimits interpersonal behavior, and it is in this

---

[1] Some lists of proposed laws and traits that would support natural law include the *Decalogue*, Thomas Aquinas (see ref. 4 below), the eight natural laws of C. S. Lewis in his book, *The Abolition of Man* (Oxford, 1943), and, for primitive society, see: J. F. Johnston, Jr., *Natural Law and the Rule of Law*, the Philadelphia Society, 2003. The United Nations released its *Declaration of Human Rights* in 1948 listing thirty articles (rights) from which thirty wrongs can be deduced. Separate but related are lists of traits that can be considered conducive to identification of human laws consistent with the functioning of natural law: the virtuous traits of Charles Darwin (see: *The Descent of Man, and Selection in Relation to Sex*, London, 1874, 2nd edition, chapters 4 and 5), the seven "goods" identified by Dr. John Finnis (*Natural Law and Natural Rights*, Oxford, 1980), and the list of sentiments by Dr. James Q. Wilson (see ref. 3 below).

arena that its role in governance is revealed. Through the mechanism of one's conscience, it provides a common moral base for social interactions among all people and thereby stabilizes communal existence. It is not relevant to all individual behavior, which is otherwise unabridged. It also is not a "social contract" meant to guide a society in a specific direction, a contract that would invite endless theorizing about what a perfect society might be and what methods should be imposed to attain perfection. It is instead a protection for those who might be victims of those who choose to ignore natural law, perhaps even attempting to impose their ideas of perfection on you. There would be few laws necessary were everyone to follow the guidance of natural law, for there would be no fear of theft or bodily harm coming from others. There would, of course, be allowance for differences of opinion, but authoritarianism would theoretically be nonexistent except for the authority of agreed-upon laws (*e.g.*, traffic laws) that would necessarily have penalties for disobeying. But to be practical, human nature is such that there will never be a shortage of transgressions of natural law, so coercion will be required to (1) protect individuals from transgressions of their natural rights, (2) defend/assist the victim of transgression, and (3) prevent the expansion of a transgress, especially to the point that an expanding association can establish its own positive laws inimical to natural law, *i.e.*, to individual liberty, and ultimately to dominate it.[2]

Natural law may exist, but what of it?

What is the proof that natural law exists? (1) There is a commonality in certain human social interactions across all societies that is consistent with an innate moral system, one that, underneath a panoply of positive laws and other social directives, does not vary with regard to the status of disparate individuals, societies and civilizations.[3] (2) There is a theological and philosophical support for the existence of natural law insofar as human reason has been considered designed for its implementation and has been assigned both the ability and the responsibility of identifying its components and following its direction.[4] (3) It is claimed that proof of natural law is self-evident, an analytic position not requiring proof. (4) A similar approach is based on contradiction; if in inversion of a law is absurd, then the original version can be true. (5) It has been proposed that natural law evolved in humans by the supposedly proven mechanism of Darwinian evolution. The first of these proofs can be considered both scientifically and statistically supportable, and in fact it is considered so by many.

But even if human reason is sufficient to prove that natural law exists or if theories attached to Darwinian evolution in time become incontrovertible facts, there needs to be a determination as to *why* it exists. There is no *a priori* reason to consider natural law as beneficial, for, if such an assumption is made, natural law outside the realm of theology becomes a philosophical invention, as all that relates to it is deductive. And if we can find no reason for its existence, it is of no more significance than, for example,

---

[2] Positive laws are those statutory laws made by human agencies.

[3] James Q. Wilson, *The Moral Sense*, New York, 1993. Dr. Wilson does not use the term "natural law" in his book, but separately he has stated that he hopes the moral sense and natural law are equivalents.

[4] Paul E. Sigmund, *St. Thomas on Politics and Ethics*, New York, 1988, pp.48-50.

the Goethe bone.[5] If twenty unrelated cultures are studied and sixteen recognize the equivalent of natural law or the Golden Rule, this would indicate with high probability that natural law is integral to all societies. On the other hand, statistical proof of its presence does not mean that it is worthwhile. Margaret Mead, who characterized natural law as a "species-specific capacity to ethicalize," was sufficiently convinced of natural law as a proven phenomenon to affirm that, based on her experience, its presence was felt in every primitive society.[6] But the dismal lifestyle and brutishness of most primitive societies are no proof that natural law is a good thing. It is, of course, commonly understood that expressions of natural law are easily overcome or ignored by human laws, greed, social pressure and the like. But this argument is an assumption, not proof. Perhaps natural law merely represents the aggregate consequence of random genetic change or founder effect in our ancient ancestors. To determine why natural law exists, some characteristic of society that depends on and coexists with it needs to be analyzed, its usefulness or hinderance to society determined, and a causal relation thereby shown.

The purpose of natural law

It is possible that identifying the true purpose of natural law is impossible or is even forbidden to human knowledge. For purpose of discussion, however, let us presume it is a secular Eden that might result from free rein of human ingenuity. But that ingenuity would be manifested in bits and pieces of all kinds and dimensions of knowledge, its consequences unpredictable at the time of each discovery, and thus the final product would not have been an intended product. In a completely free society and given the broad spectrum of ideas of humans on just about everything they come upon, the range of possibilities that would promptly result from the discoveries and inventions of that society is enormous. How then can the secular purpose for natural law be recognized?

As an opening statement, in an authoritarian society the role of natural law is subservient to positive laws, if the former is allowed to make its existence felt at all, and it is the positive laws and those who promulgate them that will direct society. In contrast, a characteristic of natural law is its dissuasion of an individual from infringing on the rights of others; axiomatically, there is no constraint on actions so long as they do not infringe on the rights of others.[7] Discovery, invention and open discussion prevail. As this applies to all persons, it provides a justification for a free and open society that will effectively direct itself, will progress even if we at the moment do not know what that direction is. Society acting in concert with natural law would be truly democratic, although not in the restrictive political sense of majority rule. Can all this be shown?

The concept of natural law promoted in this monograph must be compared to other concepts of natural law that focus on ways to legally regulate society and social morality, *i.e.*, natural law implementation as positive law. This attempt at implementation involves devising laws consistent with contemporary opinions about the role of natural law and the appropriateness of positive laws. But if the idea that natural law is to be

---

[5] Goethe bone, the "incisive," or "intermaxillary bone" in humans, is found in many mammals, and, while a curiosity of anthropology, is of little clinical interest.

[6] Margaret Mead, *Some Anthropological Considerations Concerning Natural Law*, in *Natural Law Forum*, 1961, paper 59, pp. 51-64; http://scholarship.law.nd.edu/nd_naturallaw_forum/59.

[7] See Exursus 6 for a more extensive treatment of this general interpretation of natural law and its association with the Ten Commandments and the Golden Rule.

expressed by no transgression of another's natural rights as its essence, then the transference of details of natural law to society's regulatory and legislative systems is either unnecessary or inappropriate, for the correct venue of natural law is within the individual, not a society's legal system. The answer to this dilemma is not to implement details as to what popular opinion considers is consistent with natural law, but simply to *minimize those laws that infringe on natural rights*. Seen in this light, natural law serves more as a "bill of rights" protection for the individual. All this sounds familiar.

There can, of course, be laws for punishing such crimes as are recognized by a society, *e.g.*, running a red light, and inevitably among those crimes will be natural law infractions. But the legal implication of the "bill of rights" role of natural law is limited to protection of, not granting of, the individual liberty implied in, and required by, natural law. It is not to be involved in deciding punishment for infractions of natural law. Punishment of the guilty is a separate issue and one to be managed as a community, in that the primary purpose of punishment is to prevent future such bad actions from affecting other members.

The relevance of the preceding to the present topic can now be resolved. One proof of the existence of natural law, as interpreted above, would be to show whether individual liberty is harmful, not a threat, or a benefit to society. If individual liberty is indeed a requirement for natural law to convey social benefits, then a "free" society should fare well and an "unfree" society should not. The more consistent this finding among human societies the firmer would be the proof. Furthermore, as natural law is considered embedded in every individual, one should expect its benefits (1) to proceed not from a special group of individuals within a society but throughout society, and (2) to benefit all members of society. Benefits should emanate throughout society regardless of one's status or privilege. Those benefits may be difficult to differentiate from beneficial events that might happen by chance or by authoritarian design, and it may even be difficult to identify what exactly is meant as a beneficial event. Furthermore, that event may be evanescent, permanent, minor, major, or even undetectable for the moment. It is necessary, however, that the proof of natural law beneficence be assessable through quantifiable objective effects. Allowances would have to be made for contemporary competing events, both positive and negative, for they might alter the perceptibility of a beneficial or detrimental effect attributable to natural law.

Existential justification for attributing beneficence to natural law

One measure that would fulfill a basic requirement as a gauge of beneficence is life expectancy. For all societies, both an appreciation of living and a fear of dying contribute to a thankfulness for a longer life and for relief when saved from a life-threatening experience, thus broadening the scope of the presumed beneficence of a longer life and minimizing the chance that any judgment on its beneficence is merely hedonistic self-indulgence and thereby a false measure of natural law beneficence. Further support is provided by the universal desire for a longer life irrespective of status or privilege. Even those with a long life desire an even longer life. As for the method of determination of life expectancy, the society at large needs be assessed, not just those few in society who, because of special treatment, access, or protection might have a greater life expectancy than the majority of the population. Preferably, if there is a subpopulation that has special privileges that might contribute to longer life, data from that subpopulation should be excluded from any analysis of life expectancy in that society.

The Natural State of Medical Practice looked at historical and prehistorical periods of prosperity, population increase, personal freedom, and group autonomy found in the settlement hierarchy phase of a large primary city in Mesopotamia, Egypt, India, China, and Ionic Greece, and in our modern Western civilization. Remarkably, life

	Earliest increased longevity >45 years	Earliest increase longevity >baseline
China	1970	1950
India	1970	1930
Russia	1950	1930
Egypt	1960	1950
Brazil	1950	1940
Japan	1930	1910
Peru	1950	1950
Mean value	**1954**	**1937**
USA	1900	1890
UK	1905	1875
France	1900	1820
Germany	1910	1895
Sweden	1875	1825
Canada	1900	1860
Netherlands	1890	1890
Mean value	**1897**	**1865**

expectancy has increased only in the West and only in the last 150 years. Furthermore, *The Natural State of Medical Practice* provides evidence that this is attributable to recognition of natural rights for the common citizenry subsequent to the Reformation in the 16th C (see excursus 6). While this single event is not in itself a statistically strong argument supporting a beneficent natural law,[8] its significance is increased in that a longer life expectancy in the West has been followed by an increase in longevity in other regions of the world beginning about two or three generations later as shown in the above Table. In other words, it is a Western legacy, not a global inevitability.[9] This evidence of human

---

[8] It has been argued that increased longevity was also apparent in ancient Greece and Rome. For the common man and woman, however, the matter is unproven and will remain so, if for no other reason than that slavery/serfdom was common in ancient civilizations. In addition, factors other than medical discovery may have been in play, such as the safety of local drinking water or climatic rigors.

[9] By a two-tailed t-test the difference between the top and bottom mean values is significant ($p < .001$) in each column. I derived these dates from graphs available on https://www.statistica.com. As the mean value of age at death for most, if not all, past civilizations is in the range of 30-40 years (including some studies that exclude from their calculations deaths in childhood; see vol. 3 of *The Natural State of Medical Practice* for specific values), the first column is based on the specific year that mean life expectancy exceeded 45 years, *i.e.*, significantly greater than prior human experience. The second column is based on several years of increasing longevity that were followed by a consistent increase to the present day; *i.e.*, evidence that system-wide progress was occurring. A

progress, the beneficence of a longer life, can therefore be attributed to increasing civil liberty of the common citizenry and thereby a consequence of adherence to natural law, its timing suggesting the Reformation as its origin.

Another gauge of beneficence could be the number or percent of people in a society living in misery. This should logically correlate with life expectancy, but perhaps this is not so. It needs to be examined. Total population is not a measure of beneficence because longer life expectancy and improved infant mortality are important contributors to total population. Even expressions of satisfaction or dissatisfaction with contemporary affairs is inadequate. It is recorded, for example, that some persons waiting to be sacrificed in Aztec rituals refused to be saved by soldiers of Cortez. And, in the closely inhabited community of Catalhoyuk of the 8th millennium BC, evidence of change or progress over a thousand years is lacking despite an estimated life expectancy of little more than thirty years. Quantitation of happiness has been attempted in modern societies using multiple markers, but their relevance to ancient society is debatable. Even the Misery Index as devised for modern societies is inappropriate, for one of its items to be analyzed is the unemployment rate, and in ancient societies there would have been no such thing as unemployment except that due to disability.

A better gauge of beneficence is medical practice, for it, along with writing, can be a measure of societal progress. In assessing quantifiable data on medical practice as it existed in major and minor civilizations throughout history and prehistory, the presence of medical care as practiced by professionals and certified in their extant medical writings has been used in *The Natural State of Medical Practice* as a gauge of societal progress.

In this analysis the definition of progress in a society was "a *social* concept based on the awareness of improvability of the human condition." This statement may seem vague, but it is based on an acknowledgment that satisfaction and dissatisfaction coexist within societies, that at least some members of society know the difference, and, if desire is sufficiently strong (as it always is for medical care), some members will strive to improve aspects of the human condition as they see it. In other words, societal contentment is not being judged according to "what is," because this is an open invitation to personal opinion that will vary with one's position in society. It is, instead, oriented toward a judgment of "what can be," an indicator that something is unsatisfactory, and it therefore becomes an issue for free choice for every member of society as to how it can be improved.

In *The Natural State of Medical Practice*, its three volumes center around a description of the evolution of medical professionals in five ancient civilizations. Evidence for a medical practice by professionals was not found in twelve other prehistoric civilizations and proto-civilizations. It was concluded that the appearance of true medical practices (termed "the natural state of medical practice") appeared at a stage of early urbanization in some primary civilizations, a stage referred to as "settlement hierarchy," a spontaneous organizational pyramid of management that naturally evolves as nascent urbanization becomes more complex and peacefully adapts to prospering circumstances with an enlarging population. While the nature of human intercourse during these nascent periods of development of ancient population centers is incompletely known, the

---

secondary benefit to be derived from these contrasting data is the realization of how recent the beneficent flourish of human freedom has been, much being during the lifespan of many of us at the time of this publication. As an estimated 2,500 generations (a generation being defined as 20 years) have passed since the species *Homo sapiens* first appeared on Earth, a third of American population has personally observed approximately 0.1% of its course (those over 50 years of age).

circumstances surrounding this initially leaderless population of individuals were expressed in its adaptation to a new social environment that was not regulated by kinship but by commercialism. An element of endemic individual liberty and freedom of choice, appearing for the first time, permitted individuals and families to take advantage of social opportunity. Subsequently, an authoritarian centralized political structure evolved that replaced the element of freedom of choice present in the earlier settlement hierarchy. Restrictions on individual freedom and limitations on choice were imposed by those in power, one consequence being canonization of the earlier medical knowledge and its practitioners as the powerful sought to increase control over the mass of the population. The quality of medical knowledge then dramatically declined, and no new knowledge was added. It is concluded that infringements on individual liberty prevented the now subordinate municipal populations from abiding by natural law. They were deprived of opportunity for personal betterment. No further attempts to recover a "natural state of medical practice" were made. Authoritarian rule, usually associated with military conflict, then dominated the secondary civilizations that followed for many centuries. The positive association of a natural state of medical practice with freedom, supported by statistical analysis (see Appendix A of vol. 3), is strengthened further by its negative association with authoritarian civilizations.

The *Isagorial Theory of Human Progress* that has been propounded from the observations briefly summarized in these paragraphs is derived from the ancient Greek ἰσαγορία (isagoria), the term itself meaning "equal opportunity to speak freely in public assembly," with "freedom of assembly" understood. But the linchpin of the Isagorial Theory is consistent with a beneficent natural law in that freedom of the individual and of associations of individuals permitted self-betterment to improve their status in life, the evidence being an increase in life expectancy and nascent effective medical practices that would ultimately ease the misery of disease and injuries.

Natural law and human progress

It has now been shown that the initiation of human progress, assessable in the medical practices of six civilizations (including our own) and in life expectancy, can be explained as a consequence not of great men, great empires, wealth, power, an enlarging population, or miracles, but of human liberty. It is therefore considered a proof that this concurrence of progress and liberty has not been by chance (*i.e.*, all six examples of progress, out of eighteen civilizations and proto-civilizations analyzed, were associated with a degree of civil liberty or absence of a powerful political hierarchy, $p < .001$).

The weakness of the circumstantial evidence used in classifying the various civilizations is acknowledged in *The Natural State of Medical Practice* (vol. 3, p. 313), and thus the statistical significance of the analysis would benefit from more study. But it is a beginning. I have included among the six progressing civilizations our own, which was not done in the cited reference. Thus, the six include the democracies of the modern West, ancient Greek democracy, and the "settlement hierarchy" phase in the early development of selected cities of Mesopotamia, Egypt, India and China, a period of commercial development not yet made captive by centralized authoritarian political control.

Indeed, the association of human progress with liberty can even be considered inevitable, given that natural law and inherent genius reside in every person. That the association of civil liberty with the initiation of progress can be documented in only six civilizations reflects the extraordinary efficiency, power, and cunning of the authoritarian as expressed through physical and social tyranny and suppression of natural law. Further evidence of its inevitability is seen in the course of modern Western civilization: only in the West has human freedom been permitted a long survival, now two-and-a-half centuries, thereby enabling its recent generations to document a doubling of life expectancy of its inhabitants, not to mention the conveniences and security of daily life.

The absence of natural law

It was argued above that at its core, natural law is as a "Constitution" in that it protects our right to be individuals with freedom of choice. By that freedom we are permitted, as individuals, to be virtuous, for it has been stated many times that virtue can exist only in a free society.[10] But when positive law replaces conscience in human interactions, virtue is now defined by the State, and the individual's protection from infringement by others is subordinate to purposes of the State. Natural law continues to exist but, because of baser natures, poor judgment, or an emergency, it is disabled as a beneficent guide for protection of the individual. This is what transpired in the five major civilizations described in *The Natural State of Medical Practice*, with our own civilization now in the balance.

Furthermore, the history and prehistory of medicine shows that the beneficence of natural law will not only cease under authoritarian dictate but society can regress to a primitive state. That is, there seems to be a penalty for disregarding natural law, and that penalty involves not only cessation of progress but also the giving up of gains already made, a penalty profoundly apparent and unfathomably tragic during the European Dark Ages. And this is doubly troubling for some, for there may be many in a society who recognize, at one time or another, authoritarian decisions that are unconscionable in that they violate natural law. Those persons must therefore either act against their conscience or attempt reversal of the authoritarian stance, neither being a pleasant alternative. The penalty for disregarding natural law is particularly distressing in that the authoritarian fist in a society includes in its grasp society's innocents, those who recognize the error being made, those who are unable to do anything about it, those who are too young to understand the issues at hand, and those unborn who will inherit the misguided efforts of their forebears.

Conclusion

What would be the benefit to a society of a system of governance that would recognize the existence of natural law as a statement on liberty and would facilitate its observance in that society? Briefly, its proposed secular value as proven in the argument of this monograph and *The Natural State of Medical Practice* would lie in the freeing up of the ingenuity of the human species, for all individuals and associations of individuals

---

[10] Frederick Douglass (1818-1895) wrote "There can be no virtue without freedom - and no peace without justice." He viewed the U.S. Constitution as an anti-slavery document, with slavery being unconstitutional and against natural law and natural rights.

could contribute to improving the status of our species on earth.[11] Without that individual freedom, the purpose of natural law, which is to protect our natural rights, is denied and expression of ingenuity is crippled; the more expansive the authoritarianism, the fewer opportunities for ingenuity. Carried to the extreme, this can ultimately lead to (1) absence of human progress, (2) permanent relegation of humans to a feral existence, and (3) a world of unending authoritarian conflict.

By misappropriating the fruits of labor of others, limiting personal choice, and usurping the position of the individual in distributing benefits, governance ignores natural law and thereby denies natural rights, depersonalizes assistance, makes personal decision and responsibility unnecessary, and through this medium attracts the naïve, the irresolute and the opportunist and thus acquires power. Power once acquired, the individual cedes his conscience to the State, the definition of good and evil becomes the aegis of the State, and with the political efficiency of centralized control and the evil inherent in obtaining mastery over the direction of society, the good genie of our conscience, our moral sense, our natural law, will again be entrapped for generations to come and leave our progeny to suffer the penalty.

---

[11] The role of humaneness as it applies to other sentient species is a related but separate issue and is not discussed here.

EXCURSUS 4

The philosophical orientation of this excursus is an attempt to bypass the many versions and definitions of virtue over the ages and to assign to natural law that which is its due, namely the source of the freedom that permits virtue. Based on *The Natural State of Medical Practice*, it then develops a theorem: *Human progress and true virtue, as expressions of natural law, can occur only in a free society*, refers to its supporting evidence, and places its significance in today's world.

TRUE VIRTUE, A CONSEQUENCE OF NATURAL LAW

In previous excursus it was concluded that mankind's progress was impossible without human liberty and that avoidable delays in medical progress led to unfathomable suffering over millennia. To better understand the role of social environment in permitting progress, the present monograph also concerns human liberty, but the focus is now more on characteristics of the individual than of the group, the latter defined here as "a number of individuals having some unifying relationship" (Merriam-Webster). The justification is that there cannot be autonomous associations of free individuals if there are no free individuals. And it is through free individuals that the broad variety of human ingenuity is expressed, whereas in authoritarian states that expression is diminished. The issue is approached herein at a most general and basic level, *i.e.*, by considering the original endeavors at progress. The subsequent political implementation, intricacies and implications are complex far beyond the present subject.[1]

Natural law has been equated with conscience in our ability to distinguish between good and evil and thus how to be good and to avoid evil. In *The Natural State of Medical Practice* it was shown that, at its core, natural law is a statement on the inviolability of human liberty.[2] The connection between individual freedom and the distinction between good and evil is central to this monograph.

To begin, if the definition of "moral" involves the distinction of good from evil, definitions will vary from society to society. But natural law is understood to already incorporate the ability to make that distinction and it applies to every human, regardless of society or status. Thus, natural law should itself define morality. If this is so, the issue of cultural relativity of morals is irrelevant, because adherence to natural law becomes the definition of "moral," *i.e.*, if a person's action is consistent with natural law, the distinction between good and evil is realized and that action is morally excellent. If the action is inconsistent with natural law, that action is immoral.

Furthermore, it may sometimes be unnecessary to even consider the motive for choosing "good" over "evil" inasmuch as natural law does just that: besides being assumed to be "good," it has been *proven* to be good in that it is beneficial to human progress (see Excursus 3). In other words, good consequences of a person's action within

---

[1] A most thorough statement on freedom, natural law, natural rights, and virtue as they relate to practical implementation can be found in Thomas G. West's *The Political Theory of the American Founding: Natural Rights, Public Policy, and the Moral Conditions of Freedom*, Cambridge, 2017.
[2] See *The Natural State of Medical Practice*, especially vol. 3, chapter 12. There are also my summaries of the discussion of natural law in Excursus 2 (*A Personal View of Natural Law: Likening Natural Law to Human Autonomy*) and Excursus 6 (*Natural Law, the Ten Commandments and the Golden Rule Compared*).

a community can be independent of motive as long as that action is consistent with natural law.[3] In contrast, an inadvertent action or one with an intended good motive but inconsistent with natural law may lead to a bad consequence. In this respect natural law would seem to be efficiently self-regulating by some intrinsic mechanism no matter how it is made manifest. Either there is an assumption built into natural law (*i.e.*, the nature of natural law itself) such that, given the proper social environment, only a good, or "moral," result will ultimately emerge (the "immoral" ultimately failing), or that the role of personal judgment, such as the individual reasoning as suggested in Kant's "good will," is relatively insignificant for its operation.[4] **For such a far-reaching yet forgiving mechanism to exist within us it must be very important indeed, for it suggests that people in a society will inevitably improve their condition if nothing keeps them from obeying natural law.** Indeed, progress in that society will evolve like other natural phenomena unless disrupted by natural law transgressions, just as humans wonderfully mature as the years pass unless impeded by disease. [5] These rather astonishing statements will seem not so far-fetched as an analysis of the Isagorial Theory of Human Progress as proposed in *The Natural State of Medical Practice* (volume 1) unfolds.

A related phenomenon concerns virtue, for virtue might cohabit with natural law, and it has often been stated that without freedom there can be no virtue because authoritarian governance, in suppressing freedom, arrogates the definition of virtue to its convenience.[6] The consummate example of this is China, where, in a continuation of 4,000 years of totalitarian rule at the provincial and state level, the greatest virtue, as promulgated in its present "law-morality amalgam," remains a fervent nationalistic dedication to the authoritarian state despite its profound limitations on freedom.[7]

There are wide-ranging conceptions of virtue, including Aristotle's twelve virtues, each being the mean between two extremes (with the extremes lacking virtue), the Stoics' prudence, temperance, courage and justice, Aquinas' theological virtues of faith, hope and charity, Dante's combination of the preceding two (i.e., seven virtues), Kant's "moral strength of a human being's will in fulfilling his duty," and Nietzsche's

---

[3] A related issue is the virtue of assistance and self-sacrifice for another person in need. Such humane actions are always considered virtuous, even in wars and on opposing sides. They are recognized in The Golden Rule in that (1) they help protect the life and property of the individual in distress and (2) the proffered assistance is something we would want were we in a similar situation. While this monograph is more a fundamental description of virtue and natural law, the virtue of natural law would apply to such individual acts of humaneness.

[4] See translation by H. J. Patton of Kant's "Groundwork of the Metaphysic of Morals" in *The Moral Law*, London, 1964, chapter 1, p. 61*ff.*

[5] Another implication of natural law as portrayed in this paragraph is expressed in the question, *How did it get there?* However one might answer that question, the purpose of natural law is our betterment. Mankind's survival will inevitably follow (see conclusion of Excursus 10, *On Eden*). Furthermore, that betterment may be in the future, perhaps far in the future, which, to humans, is unknown. We are preparing for something, but what? Other animals may care for their young and travel in peaceful herds over tens of thousands of years, but natural law works daily to improve mankind's meaningful existence on earth; our survival, with its operational mechanism of ingenuity, is a separate matter. See p. 161, Ingenuity and natural law: linked in freedom.

[6] Frederick Douglass (1818-1895) wrote "There can be no virtue without freedom - and no peace without justice." He viewed the U.S. Constitution as an anti-slavery document, with slavery being unconstitutional and against natural law and natural rights.

[7] Lin, D, Trevaskes, S., *The Ideology and Institutions of China's Political-Legal System*, in *Asian Journal of Law and Society*, 6:41-66, 2019.

distinction between moralities of the master and the slave. But more simply and succinctly, Merriam-Webster, in its definition (1a), equates virtue with morality, and in definition (1b), as "a particular moral excellence." Consistent with the assertion that the complexity of an issue is directly proportional to the length of its definition, for purposes of this monograph virtue is understood to be "moral excellence." [8]

It can be asked whether virtue has any function outside of natural law. It does if a society defines it so. Even extermination of another society might be viewed as virtuous if an authoritarian regime declares it necessary and if members of that society agree or can be made or enticed to agree. But this becomes irrelevant if we assign true virtue to one thing, and one thing only, adherence to natural law.

Natural law, viewed as the equivalent of the Ten Commandments (the Decalogue) and the Golden Rule rather than an inconsistent list of "things not to do," can be considered essentially a definitive statement on individual liberty, for its restrictions advise no unwelcome interference with the life of another person.[9,10] If true virtue is defined as moral excellence and if morality is defined by natural law, promoting and defending individual liberty is virtuous. Doing something that interferes with another's liberty (against that person's will) is not virtuous and is immoral. Helping to preserve another's liberty (upon request) is virtuous and moral. Human liberty, therefore, is the *modus operandi* of natural law and is necessary for expression of true virtue (moral excellence). That such a profound statement can be attributed to something as vaguely perceived as natural law may seem unwarranted in that its importance seems inversely proportional to its phantom-like nature. In the absence of deducing specific laws that are considered to comprise natural law (as has been done in the past), how can this be applied to the human condition?

In *The Natural State of Medical Practice,* the essential role of freedom in procuring progress for the benefit of mankind was revealed. From the very origin of medical practice the relief of human suffering and averting of (premature) death have been purposefully chosen humane goals of medical care in that external threats to

---

[8] This is not the same as "*a* virtue is understood to be *a* moral excellence," for the list of specific virtues is long, each one presenting an issue with subjectivity. But what if virtue is not in partnership with natural law and is a "stand alone" phenomenon. For example, there is the subject of virtue ethics, one that has close ties with Western legal systems. There is, however, a distinction between the noun virtue and the adjective virtue of virtue ethics. Ethics has been divided into three broad categories: those in which actions are to be gauged by their good consequences, those in which actions are to be gauged by how dutifully they are fulfilled, and the nature of the character of those involved in the doing. As it concerns the latter, the legal ramifications of virtue ethics are broad, arbitrary as to motive (who defines or quantifies what is virtuous?), and, to some, paramount. Virtue ethics is not a topic of this monograph.

[9] Paul Sigmund, in *St. Thomas Aquinas on Politics and Ethics* (New York, 1988, paperback, pp.48-50), lists the following "internal expressions of natural law" by Aquinas: good is to be done, evil to be avoided, our actions should be guided by reason, we should not harm others, we should not kill others, we should not commit adultery, we should not take from others.

[10] The Golden Rule, as expressed in Mathew 7:12, is "Do unto others what you want them to do to you." Here is a version in Greek from the 2nd C AD: πάντα ουν ὅσα ἐὰν θέλητε ἵνα ποιῶσιν ὑμῖν οἱ ἄνθρωποι, οὕτως καὶ ὑμεῖς ποιεῖτε αὐτοῖς· οὗτος γάρ ἐστιν ὁ νόμος καὶ οἱ προφῆται. Literal: "everything therefore whatever you wish that they should do to you the men (the people), thus you do to them; for this is the law and the prophets." And see Excursus 6 for a more definitive discussion of the similarities of natural law, the Ten Commandments and the Golden Rule.

existence and to well-being were moderated.[11] Using a decrease in human suffering and an increase in life expectancy as incontestable "goods," therefore, statistical analysis of data in *The Natural State of Medical Practice* provides positive evidence of human goodness as a manifestation of a free society, not a society devoid of liberty.[12]

Thus, the relation of natural law and virtue can now be more broadly interpreted: virtue is not necessarily characterized as doing something for virtuous reasons. Like a moral act, it can even result from the doing of nothing that interferes with the freedom of others.[13] This is a virtuous way of life that can be looked upon as doing one's duty according to natural law. From this adherence to natural law it is obvious that one should not take or harm another person's life or property. From murder and theft to abuse and prevarication, all this is subsumed under the category of interference with the freedom of others. We are all virtuous if we do not do these things, and thus it seems axiomatic that virtue is an expression of natural law and being virtuous is our natural state and to purposely interfere with the freedom of others is an acquired aberrancy. When we interfere with freedoms of someone else, we, like taking a bite from the fruit of the Tree of Knowledge of Good and Evil, are assuming we are justified in usurping the natural right of the victim to direct his or her own life; we, intentionally or not, have become, like God, illicit arbiters of what will befall the victim of our transgression.

But what about virtuous behavior such as courage, generosity, self-control, modesty, forgiveness, kindness, humility, obedience, loyalty, sincerity, and patriotism, to list but a few examples? By present discussion, they all could be virtuous if their end is to protect another individual's autonomy (assuming that autonomy does not infringe on someone else's rights). But if their end is to interfere with that autonomy, including their life, liberty, and pursuit of happiness, they are not virtuous. Obedience, courage, and loyalty to a gang involved in smuggling people and drugs are not virtues. Even "moral excellence" can be a suspect virtue in that there have been societies that have engaged in ritual infanticide in the belief that threats to well-being of society can thereby be allayed. No, there is only one true virtue that cannot be warped into something monstrous, and that is to not interfere with the rights of others (unless requested or in response to obvious need, in which case courage and kindness, for example, could without qualification be called virtuous acts).[14]

What is our cue that we may be doing something not virtuous? Definitions of conscience are found in abundance around the world and throughout history, which is

---

[11] There also have been academic studies that revolve around the Democratic Peace Theory, a theory based on the contention that democracies do not war on other democracies, surely a "good," and while democracy is not the equivalent of freedom it is at the least a step away from authoritarian governance. There are critics of that theory, both theoretical and factual, but at present the dominant opinion is that the Democratic Peace Theory is reasonably supported by evidence. See: Rummel, R., *Never Again: Ending War, Democide, & Famine through Democratic Freedom*, Llumina Press, Coral Springs (FL), 2005, and Gat, A., *War in Human Civilization*, New York, 2006.

[12] *The Natural State of Medical Practice*, vol.3, Appendix A, p. 313. It has said many times that freedom is the source of all value in that it permits moral choice, but the present argument is more specific, *i.e.*, *good* moral choice and its virtuous expression.

[13] It would also be virtuous to protect others from losing their freedom or from bodily harm or personal loss. This is self-evident and is not discussed herein.

[14] An anonymous act of kindness to a person in need or of courage displayed in a rescue can occur in any society and would be an example of true virtue, for the intervention would be reversing a threat to the other person's well-being. But a similar act extended to a gang member whose purpose is to take from others merely reflects an attempt to avoid a loss of manpower.

strong evidence that there is such a thing. Although often considered equivalent to or identical with natural law, there is a debate about whether conscience is innate or acquired or both. This debate is widespread and ongoing, whereas natural law is considered innate and established. It has been shown that children approximately 8-10 years of age begin to question the correctness of propositions they hear from others, including from those most likely to instill in them particular opinions of what is good and bad, *i.e.*, their parents. This fledgling moral reasoning does not suggest conscience is entirely teachable. Instead, it suggests maturation of an innate process of searching for a way to properly identify the right answer to things. Conscience is therefore to be considered in this monograph as innate and as the mechanism by which guidance of natural law is allowed to consciously assert itself, an alternative guidance mechanism being defined through human reason (*i.e.*, thought, discourse, study).

If the preceding is so, then laws and actions that are inconsistent with natural law will, if an individual follows those improper laws or wrongly acts, prompt the conscience to express itself when the appropriate moment arrives, and that expression will be guilt. Guilt, not the contentment of innocence, helps us differentiate between the good and evil of our actions. Without the ability to feel or recognize guilt, evil will be unrecognized and unimpeded.[15] Authoritarianism, by carrot or by stick, impairs our ability to act on our sense of guilt when we are made to adhere to bad positive laws and wrongful social pressure, the tyranny of opinion. In contrast, in a free society guilt can more readily be detected, acknowledged and the problem corrected. There can, of course, be virtuous acts in an authoritarian state because natural law exists there as well and therefore could be sufficient to move an individual to act virtuously as a local or personal situation may require or permit. But in those societies/nations where natural law, in protecting natural rights, is the *rule*, progress and goodness will reign as long as external authoritarian threats to existence are blocked.[16]

Within the framework of elementary generalizations proposed in this monograph, it is claimed herewith that (1) human progress and true virtue are exclusive outcomes of human liberty, (2) protection of human liberty, and thereby our virtue and well-being, is our moral duty as well as the purpose of natural law.[17]

The relevance of this to *The Natural State of Medical Practice* is thus:

---

[15] "Lack of conscience" is part of the definition of a sociopath.

[16] It is obvious that political authoritarianism comes in degrees, and its susceptibility to immorality therefore does the same. Nevertheless, this monograph presents an "all or none" picture of authoritarianism for illustrative purposes, for to substitute "totalitarianism" for "authoritarianism" would imply limited relevance to all that is under discussion.

[17] If a person dives into turbulent water to save another's life, that act is virtuous whatever the outcome. If a person fights a dangerous brush fire that threatens a community, that act is also virtuous. If a person speaks out against political repression, that act is also virtuous. In each case the pronounced virtue is based on preservation of human life, protection of property, and protection from unjust prosecution. Thus, a great number of examples of virtue are made known to us each day, but each case reflects the importance of individual freedom, including freedom from premature death, from theft, and from injustice, all being consistent with adhering to natural law. Unavoidably, debate will be needed concerning what the boundaries are between one individual's freedom and another's freedom and between one individual's freedom and a democratic society's varied wants and infringements. The interaction between justice and necessity is another traditionally difficult area. But these can be resolved by reason. The bedrock for judgment remains natural law and its defense of liberty, in particular civil liberty.

Theorem: Human progress and true virtue, as expressions of natural law, can occur only in a free society.

Proofs of the theorem:

A. *The Natural State of Medical Practice* proves that authoritarian governance prevents maturation of progress and the authoritarian kinship prevents initiation of progress.
B. *The Natural State of Medical Practice* proves that the autonomous association of free people seeking self-betterment is the source of progress.
C. *The Natural State of Medical Practice*, using (1) a decrease in human suffering (purposefully and humanely effected through the invention of the natural state of medical practice) and (2) an increase in life expectancy as "goods," provides evidence that human goodness is a manifestation of a free society and absent in one devoid of liberty.[18]

Consequences of the theorem:

A. *The Natural State of Medical Practice* provides strong evidence that, by adhering to natural law, the liberation of the ingenuity of common man and woman explains the global dominance of Western civilization (which Excursus 17 renames as the Judeo-Christian Civilization.
B. As proposed and supported by *The Natural State of Medical Practice*, the penalty for not adhering to natural law is not merely cessation of progress but ultimately a reversion to empiric practices.
C. Humans, by natural law, are inherently good but can be made or enticed either to do evil or, by disregarding natural law, open the door to manipulation by evil. Man-made laws inconsistent with natural law (*i.e.*, contrary to a free society) are inimical to progress and to virtue and goodness.
D. Natural law provides protection for the rights of the individual, not the group, and therefore is in unqualified conflict with collectivism.
E. Natural law is the definitive statement on the inviolability of human liberty, but it exists not merely to protect the freedoms of the individual in whom its imprint resides. It is, at a deeper level, to be understood as an accommodation to human social interaction. Its principles are therefore logically to be considered universal and applicable to social interactions of institutions and government. The virtue it demands is far more than the praiseworthiness we apply to what we consider admirable qualities, admirable acts, and "good deeds" of individuals. Good governance accorded a free people allows the intended good emanating from natural law and natural rights to be expressed in progress and in virtue throughout a society. As an example, charitable giving would be unnecessary except for the unexpected.
F. The evidence that America is indeed a virtuous society based on its founding has been convincingly established by Dr. Thomas G. West.[27] Loss of the strength and idealism of the freedom expressed in its founding, which no other nation can supplant, will be a defeat for America in the contest of nations and inevitably

---

[18] Unless stolen, copied or purchased from a freer society.

will be the death knell for civil liberty around the globe for centuries to come. Will the Sovereign of all mankind dwell in Heaven or on Earth?

EXCURSUS 5

That the universe is not "unfolding as it should" is the topic of this excursus, for the history of the world is the history of the consequences of authoritarianism. There have been a few brief periods when this was not so, and supporting evidence from the history of medical practice is briefly repeated. It was, however, the post-Reformation West that saw a broad and sustained release of the ingenuity of the unprivileged population (common citizenry). This, plus a reaffirmation of the democratic alliance of physician and patient, first clearly expressed by Hippocratic physicians, brought about the profusion of medical knowledge that has led to a striking increase in life expectancy, first in the West and then globally. But the history of medical practice also clearly demonstrates the calamitous sequels to political interference, such as is occurring today. Predictable consequences to modern medicine are detailed.

CONSEQUENCES OF A FAILURE TO LEARN THE LESSONS OF HISTORY

The previous monograph, summarizing evidence presented in *The Natural State of Medical Practice*, discussed its relevance in today's world as objective evidence that human progress and virtue emerge from principles on which human liberty are based, the concepts of natural law and natural rights. But the relevance to today's political theater need not rely on that philosophical justification. Indeed, while the data and analyses can even be considered objective evidence for the existence of natural law, the fact is, human liberty works. The objective evidence can be viewed either theoretically or pragmatically.[1]

With the preceding in mind, the relevance of *The Natural State of Medical Practice* lies in its historical and prehistorical evidence that the course of human history has been dominated, indeed absolutely controlled, by authoritarian forces. Thus, in contrast to the optimistic "And whether or not it is clear to you, no doubt the universe is unfolding as it should,"[2] human history can be viewed as perverse and distorted as it has unfolded, and, if nothing changes the authoritarian comportment of the forces that continue to control it, that perverted manifestation will continue, perhaps as long as the human species is to exist.

But it so happens that the force to be discussed now is not represented in the annals of those who have done the dominating or in the stories and historical works that reflect select scenes from a world that is the product of the dominators. We consider here that other unwritten fact sheet of history, the dominated force, the unprivileged, the common man and woman. That there is such a force is not a fantasy, as *The Natural State of Medical Practice* has shown. To view history as an inevitable sequence of power grabs

---

[1] Here we tread on the contentious subject of historicism, which is treated briefly in *The Natural State of Medical Practice* (vol. 3. p. 299). The question is whether we can justifiably base present-day political decisions on analyses of causation derived from the study of history. To this it can be responded that the concept of human liberty is so basic that the complexity and unpredictability that may be found in related issues are insufficient to alter conclusions based on the concept of liberty alone.

[2] From the *Desiderata* of Max Ehrmann, 1927.

is to have a superficial grasp of the forces available for shaping the course of human events. It is like reading Tolstoy's *War and Peace* as an aristocratic soap opera.

There have been glimpses in human history of an underlying force waiting to be released, the story of the common citizenry, that has barely been recognized but is of such power that it has recently catapulted the West into intellectual dominance of the world. *The Natural State of Medical Practice* reveals its presence in the field of medicine. Other glimpses include (1) rare individuals who have somehow managed to emerge from the dominated population in authoritarian societies, (2) common citizens from the early urbanization settlement hierarchies of Mesopotamia, Egypt, India, China, and pre-classical Greece, and (3) from the West beginning in the 16th century.[3] It was at those six times that the "force" of the common citizenry, rather than being displayed in physical conflict against tyranny (always unsuccessful) or in a revolutionary power struggle (and merely replacing one tyrant with another), began to emerge from the shadows, or contemporary political *tabula rasa*, as a force unto itself capable of affecting the course of their respective civilizations. In medicine, the evidence for this assertion is found in those medical writings traceable to the formative years of all six civilizations:

1. Sumer – *Treatise of Medical Diagnosis and Prognosis*
2. Egypt – *Papyrus Ebers; Smith papyrus*
3. India – *Charaka Samhita*
4. China – *Huang Ti Nei Ching Su Wen*
5. Greece – *Corpus Hippocraticum*
6. Modern West – Medical journals

Medical practitioners have always been drawn from the realm of the unprivileged. But despite their characterization as illiterate and uninformed factional followers of the rich and powerful on the political stage, the phantom-like power of common men and women now has, through its creation of sophisticated medical care in the West, produced a sustained global source of beneficence to humanity, in contrast to the rare, selective, and transitory beneficence of powerful authoritarian agencies throughout history. The attribution of beneficence to those in power or to the Age of those in power or to uniquely gifted aristocratic forebears has been, in great part, a false attribution in which those who dominate (and their admirers) claim responsibility for the occasional genius arising in their midst or they praise works of genius of their prominent comrades while the dominated multitude is prevented from exhibiting any genius of its own, *i.e.*, by hobbling the opposition the elite win the prize and justify their continued political domination as an elite class.

But genius and ingenuity are evenly spread throughout humankind, indeed dwell in every individual, authoritarian and pedestrian alike, so there will inevitably be some ideas or discoveries within authoritarian circles. But there are two indisputable and overwhelming challenges to the supposed superiority of an elite class. One is simply numerical: if the mass of a civilization is free, the number of persons who can apply their ingenuity to problems at hand is far greater than those holding power. The other is also mathematical: two heads are better than one. Thus, in a free society the opportunity to

---

[3] A "snippet" list of notables from "unprivileged" backgrounds is provided on the opening page of *Medical Practice and the Common Man and Woman: A History* (Xulon Press, 2020), an abridgement of the three-volume *The Natural State of Medical Practice* (Liberty Hill Publishing, 2019).

organize into autonomous groups to solve problems relevant to self-betterment is immensely greater than bureaucratic commissions or diktats. Furthermore, efficiency, cooperation and honesty will more often favor the efforts of the former, whereas boredom, laziness, self-aggrandizement, disinterest and notoriety are some of the problems that will plague the latter. The argument of this paragraph is so obvious that it defies reason why, given a choice, anyone would prefer an authoritarian world to one based on human liberty.

And so we can now face the issue of maintaining the freedom of the common citizenry going forward. If it is maintained the answer is easy: despite its continual squabbles and zig-zag course, progress and improvement of the human condition will continue. But if their freedom disappears as centralization of political and economic power continues under the aegis of an elite political class, what will be the course of human events henceforth?

In answering this question, prehistory can be ignored unless new evidence is discovered, for the critical problem in prehistory was the inability to *initiate* progress. We must instead briefly revisit the social changes chronologically associated with *cessation* of medical progress in those four civilizations where documented medical progress was initiated:

1. Mesopotamia – Rational Sumerian medicine first appeared during early urbanization, *ca*. 2900 BC. Subsequent centralization of monarchical power, begun by Akkadian conquerors (2350 BC – 2100 BC) continued through Persian rule (550-330 BC), diluting the initially rational Sumerian contents in the extant *Treatise of Medical Diagnosis and Prognosis* with numinous practices devoid of rational medicine as edited in the 11th C BC.

2. Egypt – Predynastic Hierakonpolis, a relatively small city, is proposed as the site of medical knowledge found in the *Papyrus Ebers*. It became less important with the onset of Dynastic Egypt (*ca*. 3000 BC) where, under pharaonic rule, rational medical knowledge previously acquired was canonized and restricted to a pharaonic priesthood. No new intrinsic medical knowledge would appear even into the Common Era.

3. India –The Indus River Valley civilization deteriorated for unknown reasons beginning about 2100 BC. Medical knowledge acquired in the Vedic Age in an early city like Mohenjo-Daro was lost except for those fragments that, altered and canonized by the Brahmin caste beginning about 500 BC, form the basis for Hinduism's Ayurvedic medicine, an inexpensive ancient empiric alternative to modern Western medicine.

4. China – The Longshan civilization (*fl.* 2500 BC) with its limited authoritarianism is proposed as the source of fragments of rational medicine that would become the *Huang Ti Nei Ching Su Wen* in the 2nd C BC. Subsequent monarchical dynasties canonized its knowledge, adding bizarre concepts as edited in the 8th C AD by Wang Bing. Despite an early 20th C effort by Dr. Sun Yat-sen to initiate modern medical training, Traditional Chinese Medicine was forced onto 20th C Chinese culture by the People's Republic of China as a cheap alternative to Western medicine.

From the above it is argued that initially productive and prosperous settlement hierarchies of early urbanizations associated with medical progress were, in two of the four instances and within a century or two, subsequently dominated for millennia by totalitarian governance. Those civilizations did not progress; they got bigger but not better, and crueler rather than kinder. The Indus River Valley and Longshan civilizations differed in that they disintegrated and would not reappear, but their medical knowledge was subsequently and similarly affected by elite Brahmins in India and imperial dictate in China. In each instance, what might have become scientific medicine reverted to simple empiricism, medical progress ceased, and life expectancy for the common man and woman remained little more than thirty years. Politically, all four civilizations remained wallowing in authoritarian mire for millennia.

What about Hippocratic medicine and the Greek experience? Athenian freedoms began to contract in the 4th C BC, and, with subjugation by the Macedonians, freedom haltingly diminished within disintegrating city-states as Rome assumed possession of region (146 BC). Thus, it was primarily the disruption of Greek civilization and its Roman conquest, rather than authoritarian canonization of medical knowledge, that led to the disappearance of Hippocratic medicine. Greek medicine was not transformed; it merely became the domain of no one and disappeared. It was the Roman Catholic Church that would provide lay practitioners in the Dark Ages. Medieval universities later would idolize and canonize Hippocratic medicine when it was rediscovered, but they did not understand it. Feudal existence in the Dark Ages was terrible beyond words for the feudal serf despite the pan-European efforts of a theocratic kinship, and life expectancy remained little more than thirty years.

We come now to the sixth civilization. The association of medical progress in the West with freedom of the individual, but especially freedom of the common citizenry, can be traced to the Reformation. That progress began to manifest itself in the latter half of the 18th C, and the explosion in medical knowledge and technology in the 19th C set the stage for our subsequent medical well-being. And this has all occurred independently of Hippocratic medicine and the Renaissance. This gift of the previously dominated class has since revolutionized medical practice, health, and longevity around the world. Could such a magnificent success be lost?

Foremost to be considered is the physician-patient relation. The Hippocratic experience in the *Corpus Hippocraticum* and especially its *Oath* attest the critical role of a democratic alliance between physician and patient. The consequence of their interaction is the initiating source of all medical progress. Everything that follows is implementation and embellishment. Even the great advances of modern medicine can be viewed as achievements of findings in the physician's office that were subsequently nurtured by capitalism. Progress in other sciences, like that of medicine, results from further investigation of discoveries and invention, but they have no equivalent to the physician-patient relation. And it is the physician-patient relation that explains why medicine in ancient Greece led the way to scientific inquiry in other areas.[4]

Impositions and infractions affecting the physician-patient relation have been identified and characterized and are not repeated here.[5] It is merely to be stated that those authoritarian impositions and infractions are many and mighty, and their mechanism of action is to limit the freedom in the physician's office of both the patient and the physician by misappropriating those freedoms for their own purposes. Here is what will happen as

---

[4] Unlike medical progress and its inhibitors and catalysts documented in *The Natural State of Medical Practice*, scientific progress in other areas has so far not been similarly analyzed. But it has been stated that, in ancient Greece, the catalyst for true scientific pursuit in other areas was Hippocratic medicine, the latter being distinctly separated from the writings of contemporary natural philosophers.

[5] *The Natural State of Medical Practice*, vol. 1, Bk. 4, chap. 4, p. 546.

the process continues today, based on the history of medical practice as interpreted in *The Natural State of Medical Practice*:

1. First, the patient will viewed less and less as a unique human being, for statistical lumping and benefit to society at large will, in committee, determine patient priority and management as physicians become, as in ancient Egypt and in fact if not in name, employees of the State.
2. Second, the capitalist economic system as it relates to medical technology will be controlled by government agencies and will promptly deteriorate; corporatism (*e.g.*, crony capitalism) will flourish and innovation, accessibility and quality of product will dramatically decline.
3. Third, like ancient Chinese medicine, convenience (economic, political) will replace scientific validity in medical decisions and disciplines.
4. Next, guidelines and algorithms will be legally enforced, just as 1st C BC Egyptian "physicians" were penalized should they not follow canonized procedures from ancient times. Few qualified individuals will enter the profession of medicine, with residual physicians working for minimum wage as they did in Russia in the 1980's, and the occasional, but inevitable, poor result associated with a departure from official recommendations will, in a jury's eyes, be a crime.
5. Recognition by physicians of unique aspects of a patient's presentation, history, or response to care will decrease in importance as the physician's personal involvement becomes less valuable because the physician's opinion will not be sought as "guidelines" are followed. We will be unprepared for the unexpected and inadequately prepared for the expected.
6. As in modern Russia, medical associations will be government commissions led by non-clinicians or, more troubling, politically oriented physicians. Medical journals will parrot governmental priorities. Clinical discovery will end as professional vetting ceases and canonization of existing knowledge occurs. Seeking friends in Washington, D. C., will overwhelm seeking truth as government grants become even more the gift of political leaders seeking popular support or afraid of controversy.
7. Politicization of the intellectual hub of the profession will guarantee that, instead of early recognition, careful consideration, and selective management of a problem, any bureaucratic response will be late, massive, costly, and wrong. Some might see the recent coronavirus pandemic (2020-2022) as an example of this.
8. Most importantly, as in modern China, good medical care for the average person, especially those in rural areas, will be unavailable because of limitations on providers, facilities, and therapies.
9. In response to (8), just as in ancient Rome and thence into the Dark Ages, those with insufficient training will continue to replace fully trained physicians, and, as a result, empirical specialists and nonscientific medical treatments will gladly proliferate locally to fill the gaps in medical care as people will, of necessity, seek help from any source.
10. Life expectancy will decrease for the common man and woman as medical care reverts to the empiric.

Evidence supporting every one of these ten predictions is present today.

But the cost of loss of freedom in the medical profession will not be the only loss. The critical nature of medical care makes it a universal gauge of the progress of mankind. The history of medicine in authoritarian hands in the past shows that when civilizations lose, or, to be more specific, when the common citizenry lose, their freedoms, progress does not just rest for a while and then gradually resume its journey toward a better life. No! Life spirals down to the wonted authoritarian level of basic human survival, medical empiricism for commoners, privilege for those in charge, and unending conflict.

A perfect example is China, where totalitarian, and often essentially kinship, rule at the state and provincial levels has placed a yoke on the common man and woman for four thousand years. The vagaries in the history of its medical institutions are described.[6] But because of recent ill-conceived notions by Western commercial and bureaucratic organizations and institutions, Chinese governance has been allowed to beg, borrow, and steal modern Western technology. Today it seems prosperous and progressive, but governance remains solidly authoritarian and will remain so. Had the West not offered a helping hand to Asia the Chinese would still exist in the 16th C world of the Ming governing a hundred million impoverished farmers who had life expectancies of thirty years. And it is to this world they will return unless (1) like other prominent civilizations in history, China satisfies its needs by conquest, or (2) it frees the common citizenry. For the moment it appears to have chosen (1).

It did not need be like this. Had the inherent ingenuity of the Asian population that became modern China been permitted natural human freedoms a century ago, China might today be a leader in progress and its beneficence for all mankind, rather than being an ungrateful recipient of the fruits of freedom of the West.

There are varying methods by which power can be ceded to central governance. From examples in the 20th C, the rhetoric of the authoritarian will justify the social egalitarian policies routinely used to cement positions of power by appealing to the justice and virtue, the "ends justify the means," of those policies. The issue of virtue is an easy one: the political elite will merely redefine virtue as that which contributes to perpetuation of the State and its policies, just as China has done. Justice also will be conveniently redefined. It will not be blind, and it will indeed be convenient.

In conclusion, the only time that freedom of the unprivileged, or common, citizenry has been permitted to endure to the point that its innate force for good could be fully appreciated and self-perpetuating has been in the West since the 18th C, and modern medical progress and increased human longevity are benefits attributable to it. The beneficence of broad-based freedom of the common man and woman is so momentous, and the event of its loss will be so catastrophic, that there would seem to be no reason to seek any other guiding principle of governance but one that permits the widest possible degree of freedom, the greatest protection of natural rights, and the least centralization of political power. But beware: in an age where rhetoric is so extravagant and its expression so amplified, suasion rather than armed conflict will be the principal means used at first to restrict our freedoms. Therefore, as quoted in *The Natural State of Medical Practice*:

---

[6] *The Natural State of Medical Practice*, vol. 1, Bk. I, chap. 5, p. 93, and vol. 3, chap. 6, p. 93.

"Open your eyes to the fearful change which has been so noiselessly affected; and acknowledge BY STANDING STILL YOU BECOME A PARTY TO REVOLUTION [*sic*]."[7]

---

[7] Richard Hurrell Froude (1803-1836), as quoted at the head of Bk. IV, chap. 4, p. 546. Hurrell Froude was the elder brother of the famous English historian, James Anthony Froude. A cleric, Hurrell's statement is to be found in *Remarks on State interference in Matters Spiritual*, in *Remains of the Late Reverend Richard Hurrell Froude*, M. A., vol. 1 of Part 2, Derby, 1839, p. 196. Although pertaining to "matters spiritual," Froude adds the comment, based on the principles of Hooker, that it "goes to any kind of State interference at all." Froude, part of the early 19th C Oxford Movement in England, was arguing a principle of 16th C Calvinism.

EXCURSUS 6

The common identity of natural law, the Decalogue and the Golden Rule is argued in this excursus, and a common interpretation is derived: Do not transgress the rights of others. An explanation for the tardy mindfulness of natural law and natural rights by mankind is offered, and the scope of their authority is extended to include government itself. It is argued that in brief periods in early urbanization before powerful political hierarchies had yet to transgress natural law there was evidence of progress in medicine, but transgression promptly intervened, and progress ceased. This changed with the 16th C Reformation because natural law and natural rights were increasingly acknowledged and, into the 17th C, natural rights were increasingly protected. Consequently, the 18th C saw the emergence of medical discovery that flourished in the 19th C, and the 20th C saw the West as the intellectual center of the world. Such was the power of complying with natural law.

NATURAL LAW, THE TEN COMMANDMENTS AND THE GOLDEN RULE COMPARED

The three subjects of this monograph, natural law, the Golden Rule, and the Ten Commandments (collectively, "Laws") are discussed in *The Natural State of Medical Practice* in the context of individual and group liberty and human progress. This would seem unexpected because the Laws are commonly considered ethical statements arising from Judeo-Christian writings, with the Ten Commandments being those cited in *Exodus* 20:2-17, natural law as explained by Thomas Aquinas (1225-1274) in his *Summa Theologica*, and the Golden Rule as stated in *Matthew* 7:12. An association of ethical issues with the politics of liberty is to be expected, but their relevance to progress of a society is not obvious. This monograph explores further the commonality of the three Laws and their relevance to progress and *The Natural State of Medical Practice*.

Each of the three ethical statements can be a lifetime study in itself, but a brief working description is desirable for those, including the author, who cannot or choose not to become students of the issues:

1. Dr. Paul Sigmund has translated works of Thomas Aquinas, and from them he has extracted a list of natural laws that include:[1]
   a. We know good is to be done, evil avoided.
   b. We know we should not harm others.
   c. We know we should not kill others.
   d. We know we should not commit adultery.
   e. We know we should not take from others.
2. The Ten Commandments have been conveniently divided into two categories, the "ritual" commandments and the "ethical" commandments.[2] The latter is more our focus here, and they are, briefly and in no particular order:
   a. You will not kill; οὐ φονεύσεις
   b. You will not commit adultery; οὐ μοιχεύσεις
   c. You will not rob; οὐ κλέψεις

[1] Paul Sigmund, *St. Thomas Aquinas on Politics and Ethics*, New York, 1988, pp.48-50.
[2] This is not a rigid distinction. See: Prager, D., *The Ten Commandments,* Washington, D.C., 2015.

d. You will not bear false witness; οὐ ψευδομαρτυρήσεις κατα τοῦ πλησίον σου μαρτυρίαν ψευδῆ

e. You will not lust after your neighbor's wife; οὐκ επιθυμήσεις τὴν γυναῖκα τοῦ πλησίον σου (or the house, the slave, handmaid, ox, ass, or anything else of your neighbor)

3. The Golden Rule is different in that it indicates in general terms not only what we should do to others but what we would like to be done to us in similar circumstances: "Therefore all things whatsoever ye would that men should do to you, do ye even so to them; for this is the law and the prophets" (Matthew 7:12, KJV). This dual admonition receives attention later, but regarding "...do ye even so to them" it is reasonable to conclude that, as we do not wish to be killed, harmed, robbed or lied to, it is implied that, as a minimum, the Golden Rule can be construed to encompass purposeful harm to others. Beyond that, it is obvious that by "the law and the prophets" is meant the Mosaic Ten Commandments.

Taking the preceding in order, evidence of natural law has in some form been documented in almost all societies, including primitive ones, and may be equated with the "moral sense" of Dr. James Q. Wilson.[3] It by definition is a body of unchanging moral principles innate in all people in all times and places and is regarded as a basis for all human conduct (derived from the Oxford English Dictionary). Treatment of natural law in *The Natural State of Medical Practice* is notable in that the "do not do" restrictions of natural law were combined in a single statement. A generalization was devised that seemed internally consistent with traditional interpretations: "We know we should not transgress the rights of another person."[4] This interpretation was then employed in explaining the inhibitory effects of coercive egalitarianism and egalitarian kinships on the evolution of primitive societies.[5] Their internally enforced equity was considered a transgression of natural rights of individual members, and it was concluded that such transgression could lead to social entrapment of a society for millennia. Natural law thus interpreted is more than just a short list of things that the individual is not to do to avoid punishment. Rather, it implies that every person has basic rights that are to be protected, in effect declaring the inviolability of human liberty. When circumstances prevailed that supported the development of cities, people exchanged the enforced equity of the tribe for the greater freedom of choice to be found in the settlement hierarchy of early urbanization.

---

[3] (1) Margaret Mead, *Some Anthropological Considerations Concerning Natural Law*, in *Natural Law Forum*, 1961, paper 59, pp.51-64; http://scholarship.law.nd.edu/nd_naturallaw_forum/59; (2) James Q. Wilson, *The Moral Sense*, New York, 1993. Dr. Wilson does not equate the moral sense and natural law in his book, but he elsewhere has stated he hoped they were the same (see Acton Institute in *Religion and Liberty*, vol. 9, No. 4, *The Free Society Requires a Moral Sense, Social Capital*).

[4] "We know that we should not kill, harm, commit adultery, or take from others" is interpreted as a general statement that includes the traditional "natural" rights of life, liberty, pursuit of happiness, and property. Specific rights, therefore, are not mentioned herein. This interpretation does not infringe on offering assistance in any form, whether or not requested.

[5] On p. 659, vol. 3, of *The Natural State of Medical Practice* the relevance of individual liberty to natural law is expressed thus: "Rather, [a person's] freedom is based on the innate understanding of other individuals around him that he is not to be kept from doing what he wants to do, just as he is not to interfere with them. Natural law has a moral orientation; it is not a legal document."

A temporary flare of human progress ensued that is confirmed in ancient medical writings.[6]

Moving now to the ethical laws of the Ten Commandments that make up its "do not do" list, the context of the Ten Commandments is broadly disputed and a relation to earlier societies proposed. There are similarities with the Code of Hammurabi, the precepts of Ma'at (preceding the Ten Commandments by two thousand years), verses in the Quran, and categories in the Yoga Sutras of Hinduism (*e.g.*, the yamas, or list of "do not do," traceable to the Rig Veda). In all cases, these lists can be considered infractions not to be imposed on others, with the specific items listed merely being the more egregious infractions. The generous interpretation of "We should not transgress on the rights of another person" seems reasonable for them as well as for natural law. An association, indeed identity, between natural law and the Ten Commandments is also recognized.[7] Thus, I would propose that any similarity between the Ten Commandments and the other ancient moral directives does indeed reflect a commonality insofar as natural law is universal, for the others are expressions of moral orientation that all humans share. But the Ten Commandments are comprehensive, specifically delineated and specifically directed. Unlike our conscience, which is easily overruled by events, the Ten Commandments are the definitive and unequivocal statement of natural law.

Finally, there is a clue to the relevance of human liberty in the Golden Rule as translated above, although it is commonly considered to be an exhortation to be kind and to help those in need. The equivalent of the Golden Rule is found in almost all societies and is often equated with natural law.[8] It is not meant as a request for others to do good things to us. The reference to what is acceptable behavior toward ourselves is used merely as an example of the kinds of actions one should do for others. But the Golden Rule, while implying a positive and virtuous action, is fraught with awkward interpretations.[9] Indeed, it is more consistent in meaning when interpreted as not to do something hurtful to another, *i.e.*, in a negative sense, the "silver" rule: "Do not do to other persons what you would not want them to do to you." But there is a way to synthesize the Golden and

---

[6] The writings and their proposed approximate dates include: Sumer (3000 BC) – *Treatise of Medical Diagnosis and Prognosis*; Egypt (3000 BC) – *Papyrus Ebers*; India (2500 BC) – *Charaka Samhita*; China (2000 BC) – *Huang Ti Nei Ching Su Wen*. See Bk. I, chapters 2-5, of vol. 1 of *The Natural State of Medical Practice* for their descriptions, significance, transitory nature, canonical alterations, and justification for the proposed dates.

[7] Martin Luther himself was clear on this point, writing in *How Christians Should Regard Moses* (1525): "For what God has given the Jews from Heaven, He has also written in the hearts of men." Also see: Randall Smith, *Thomas Aquinas on the Ten Commandments and the Natural Law*, in *The Decalogue and Its Cultural Influence*, Dominik Markl, editor, Sheffield, 2013, pp.148-168.

[8] Blackburn, S., *Ethics: A Very Short Introduction*, Oxford, 2001, p. 101.

[9] No one would suggest that the Golden Rule is meant to be a selfish rule stating we should be willing to give money or property to someone else because they might give us money or property; "I would like you to make me rich, and therefore I should try to make you rich" is an "insider trading" interpretation. Second, if it is meant that you do something helpful for others in need because you would like them to help you in similar circumstances, that can be selfish in suggesting a reason not to help someone in need if you think they wouldn't help you. Third, if it is meant to do something helpful for others because you would like to think they would do the same if circumstances were reversed, that is a highly subjective and perhaps impractical standard. It makes sense only if you assume the other persons share your valuation of the need, which is quite a jump of faith. Fourth, another interpretation is that you should go around doing good deeds for others because you would like people to do good deeds to you. This suggests a form of barter, which is not how most people interpret the Golden Rule.

silver rules that can arguably come closer to expressing the true meaning of both. That interpretation is: "I will leave you alone (unless requested) if you will leave me alone (unless requested)." From this it is understood that we will not transgress another person's rights because we would not want that person to transgress our rights (but we are there in case of need), a statement far more comprehensive than a list of things we should not do and do not want to have done to us. Its meaning is not open to misinterpretation. At the same time it is a positive statement (I will, you will) and is stating "I will not harm you."

Thus, natural law, the Ten Commandments and the Golden Rule, as interpreted in *The Natural State of Medical Practice* and this monograph share a common thread: "Do not transgress on the rights of another person." But their message has traditionally been directed at the individual. In that it follows that they apply to every citizen, should they not then extend to government? This did not happen in ancient times. A feature of the above Laws is that there is no use of a word translatable as "freedom" or "liberty" that might imply a place for implementing the ethical Laws for society as a whole. This is consistent with those ancient times, for the concept of individual liberty, much less as a political goal, would have been considered absurd.

It is understandable, therefore, that as cities grew to be grand empires, monarchical rule dominated almost without exception.[10] Their governance routinely transgressed life, liberty and property of citizens and non-citizens to accommodate those in power or their favorites. But even more important, in so doing citizens were prevented from acting in their own best interest. Thereby those discoveries and inventions that might have emanated from broad-based human ingenuity were prevented. There was a fleeting glimpse of the fruitfulness of liberty in primary cities of Sumer, Egypt, India and China, as confirmed in ancient medical writings discussed in vol. 1 of *The Natural State of Medical Practice*, but this promptly ceased.

Ancient and venerable as they are, therefore, the Laws remained a useless force beyond that conferred on interpersonal relations. If social agencies need not follow the Laws, whether interpreted traditionally or as discussed herein, what does this mean? It means that, while individual citizens have an ethical guide, governments do not. Should the government see merit in killing or the taking of the money or property of a person, citizen or non-citizen, there seems to be no historical link to the ethical Laws unless governance is to some degree controlled by a citizenry that knows it should observe those Laws, *i.e.*, such as a democracy. The ancient Hebrew tribes, while not democratic in the traditional sense, did have deliberative councils that allowed open discussion (the *edahs*, p. 86).[11] Perhaps this is a clue to the relevance of the ethical Laws to modern progress, as well as an explanation as to why it took so long for them to make a difference.

---

[10] The Indus River Valley civilization may be a remarkable exception, at least for part of its 3rd millennium BC existence, a point of discussion in vol. 3, chap. 5, p. 75, of *The Natural State of Medical Practice*.

[11] The Hammurabi law code of 1750 BC, much discussed and often admired, is such an authoritarian treatise. It describes the punishment to be imposed for a great variety of infractions that are presented in an "if-then" pattern. Any ethical aspect to the Hammurabi code represents Hammurabi's ethical point of view, not that of his subjects; he says so himself in its prologue. In contrast, the 500 BC Gortyn law code found on Crete evolved over a century or two in response to legal situations as they arose, analogous to English common law. Early steps toward democracy had already been undertaken in Greek city-states of Ionia. The definitive version of the Gortyn code, the product of a Dorian city-state, may not have been a product of a formal democracy, but its carefully thought-out revisions represent more a consensus than a dictum. See: Michael Gagarin, *The Organization of the Gortyn Law Code*, in *Greek, Roman and Byzantine Studies*, 23:129-146,

Ancient Greece was the first remarkable exception. The evolution of democracy in many Greek city-states was coincident with the appearance of effective medical practice as documented in the *Corpus Hippocraticum*. Arising in 6th C BC city-states of Ionia and given two centuries to prosper, there is a clear historical association between the success of civil liberty, as limited as it was, and the initiation of medical progress. It is properly stated that this glimpse of liberty, without historical parallel, came from a society that tentatively but bravely had decided popular control of the city-state, based on the idea that "I will leave you alone if you will leave me alone, but we must work together to survive" was superior to rule by a monarch or tyrant, and it permitted personal investment in decisions on governance. Intentionally or not, natural law was being implemented. Whereas it is proposed that four primary cities of the civilizations of Mesopotamia, Egypt, India, and China and the freedoms of their "settlement hierarchy" phases developed *de novo* during early urbanization and prior to their monarchies, Greek democracies developed in spite of preexisting monarchies, oligarchies, and tyrannies, although Miletos, the proposed city of origin of Hippocratic medicine, was settled as a primary city-state, *ca.* 1100 BC. The Greek political choices, while contested and incompletely implemented, were based on common sense and recognition that the same rational intelligence they knew to be part of their own psyche must also abide in their neighbor, and it must be met on equal terms and acknowledged rather than subdued. In this relatively open and "free" environment poor itinerant medical practitioners began to settle in cities, associate, and pool their knowledge.[12] Thus, the connection between the ethical Laws and human progress was tentatively confirmed. Sadly, this lasted only two centuries.[13]

We now come to the climax of this monograph, our own time. It remained to the 16th C Reformation in the West to demonstrate that the underlying message of the Laws would release a force that would propel the West to intellectual leadership of the world, that force being its common citizenry as they arose from feudalism.

The fracturing of the pan-European doctrinal kinship of the Roman Catholic Church precipitated by the actions of Martin Luther was superseded by calls for religious freedom. The concept of individual freedom within and without a "church" was then debated and its philosophical justification sought in biblical contexts. Foremost in Reformation thought on morality was the Ten Commandments. By the 18th C laws more broadly interpreted as "Do not transgress on the rights of another person" were constraining the role of governance over the lives of average citizens. Slowly the West saw its governments introduce democracy and ethical tenets into laws respecting the rights of citizens, thereby protecting them from murder, theft and fraud perpetrated or permitted by the government itself. This change in institutional prerogatives increasingly tolerated personal expressions of freedom and self-interest that ultimately led to the rise of the West in less than two centuries (late 18th C to the late 20th C).[14] With the removal

---

1982, Univ. of Texas, Austin, although a more complete exposition of texts from Crete is found in *The Laws of Ancient Crete*, Oxford, 2016, by the same author.

[12] Several important Hippocratic treatises are translated literally and in the vernacular in vol. 2 of *The Natural State of Medical Practice*.

[13] Book II of vol. 1 of *The Natural State of Medical Practice* is devoted to the Grecian saga.

[14] I do not accept the suggestion that colonial dominance was the cause of intellectual prominence in the West. Medical practice, printing of books and journals, scientific discovery and relevant new industries were not products of colonialism. If anything, colonialism was a state-sponsored enterprise of a mercantile nature, not an intellectual one. It was a search for wealth rather than a

of the authoritarian thumb on the common citizenry unbelievable progress in longevity, comfort, moderation of illnesses, invention, and discovery has brought us to the pinnacle of human progress where we now find ourselves.[15]

This remarkable success did not occur because specific laws were written that favored the physician, the scientist, and the botanist. Nor were they written so as to prohibit murder, robbery, injury, fornication, and prevarication. In fact, the latter may have worsened civilization-wide because some would confuse liberty with license. But the laws that evolved which saw the release of the ingenuity of the unprivileged man and woman that led to modern progress were laws protecting their natural rights.[16] Had the specific "do not do" ethical laws alone been enacted but the governance remained authoritarian, people might have been protected by a police state, but the price would be (1) no protection of natural rights and (2) ethical laws as defined by the State in the manner of Hammurabi. This trade-off of freedom for security would have been a very bad decision and progress would have been impossible. Instead, with an increasingly democratic society the laws came to reflect the extent to which both citizen and State appreciated the same ethical goal, one that recognized the morality of the Ten Commandments and the validity of civil liberty. The full import of individual liberty and autonomous associations of a free people soon followed.

The purpose of natural law discussed so far has been to preserve the natural rights of the individual from predation from either another individual or the State. But progress itself is the product of autonomous groups (koinons).[17] It has been argued that the brief periods of medical discovery during early urbanization in Sumer, Egypt, India, China, and Greece were the work of groups, not a single individual.[18] Does the protection of natural rights also apply to groups, *i.e.*, do an individual's natural rights justify a similar protection for groups?

Perhaps the role of natural law in a group or institution depends in part on the number of individuals involved. The more individuals involved, the autonomy of the individual member tends to decrease, and the group tends to acquire an authoritarian face. I am unaware of any studies relating authoritarianism to group size alone, but it is clear

---

source of knowledge or mechanism of progress. It would have occurred with or without the Reformation and represented authoritarian thinking, not the popular mind. Indeed, it was well under way long before the Reformation.

[15] Capitalism has also been a contributor to Western dominance, but as discussed in vol.1, pp. 199 and 548, capitalism was not a factor in the development of scientific medicine; *i.e.*, true capitalism (entrepreneurial, not mercantile or state capitalism), like the profession of medicine, was a consequence, not a cause, of civil liberty. But it contributed greatly to the spread of rational medicine, especially through books and journals.

[16] A most thorough statement on freedom, natural law, natural rights, and virtue as they relate to practical implementation can be found in Thomas G. West's *The Political Theory of the American Founding: Natural Rights, Public Policy, and the Moral Conditions of Freedom*, Cambridge, 2017.

[17] The koinon (κοινόν), or voluntary automatous group pursuing a common self-interest, is described in vol. 1 of *The Natural State of Medical Practice* and is proposed as the source of medical knowledge found in the Hippocratic *Corpus*. The common dictum, "two heads are better than one," is the basis for the superiority of the group over the individual in promoting progress, although today progress can more easily result from a single individual's invention or discovery because of the interaction of communication tools, media, and economics that can influence consumers far afield and speed success. For a definition of group as used herein see pp. 17 and 155, "A group discussion."

[18] Discussion on this point is found in vol. 1 of *The Natural State of Medical Practice*.

that the social dynamics of a small autonomous group differ from a large association in more than scale. The former is freely entered into and easily left if there is disagreement. Personal opinions of each member can be readily and fully expressed and debated. There is little penalty to the individual and no infringement on natural rights.

For large associations, however, membership usually has as its motive some personal advantage that relies on the power of that association, and that motive often is security. In obtaining that advantage some loss of individual freedom will be the trade-off. For corporations, the same applies. Thus, the larger the group the more akin it is to a government unto itself, especially today. Its own survival supersedes that of its individual members, and its power becomes a bargaining chip when interacting with government (corporatism). In this sense, therefore, it should be up to the membership to identify within the larger group its protections for natural rights. The most immediate response to infringements would be to look for another job, although this merely provides an opening to hire a person who is sympathetic to the cause of the larger group. This is separate, of course, from rules or regulations specific to the functions of large associations or corporations. But the principal point is that boundaries on natural rights/laws of individuals within a large organization can be debated or declined. With the State, however, there is little choice.

So we come to the underlying meaning of the three Laws representative of Judeo-Christian morality in the sense that they sanction freedom from unwelcome interference in our personal decisions, whether by individuals, groups, or the State. In a summing of traditional interpretations, their deeper meaning is that individual liberty is first and foremost to be protected not by laws against specific infractions but by protection of natural rights. That meaning has been succinctly expressed by Dr. Randy E. Barnett: "The purpose of natural law is to preserve our natural rights."[19] He also points out that natural rights govern how others should act toward natural rights holders, not how rights holders should act to others. The latter is the role of natural law. The larger the group, greater can be the impetus for restriction of natural rights, both for its members and for its competition. Still, this can be debated and declined. Unfortunately, with the State and centralization of political power infringements are more difficult, more important, and harder, if not impossible, to exit or decline. Big government is the biggest problem.

In conclusion, natural law, the Ten Commandments, and the Golden Rule, as interpreted and contextually analyzed in *The Natural State of Medical Practice*, are revealed to be (1) equivalent in meaning, (2) universal statements and a moral code based on the inviolability of human liberty, (3) a mandate for civil liberty for every individual, and (4) indispensable for human progress. The Laws have been available to promote human progress for thousands of years. Their domain and popularity have been prodigious, but, in the hands of the authoritarian, so has their fragility. Let us not forget this today.

---

[19] See Dr. R. E. Barnett, *A Law Professor's Guide to Natural Law and Natural Rights*, in *Harvard Journal of Law & Public Policy*, 1997, summer issue.

EXCURSUS 7

A description of mankind's natural aversion to crowding as displayed by primitive nomadic and sedentary groups opens this excursus. Manifested in small groups by early humans for social contact and protections centering around family, it is proposed that larger and thereby more authoritarian kinships were preferentially avoided except for safety. In rare but remarkable instances the repressive early tribal kinship was abandoned for commercial urbanization, although ensuing progress would, within a few centuries, be blocked by authoritarian political governance. This is a warning that the ethic of natural law encounters increasing risk of subversion as population density increases and we lose or cede our natural rights and responsibilities to a politicized central governance. Should this occur the consequence will be perennial conflict and regression of progress already obtained. Would that it were possible to safely disperse.

HUMAN DISPERSION AND NATURAL LAW; GOVERNMENT AS A KINSHIP

It is repeatedly claimed that man is a political animal,[1] and there are studies of chemical mediators that affect individual human interactions with things, events, and other humans.[2] The latter approach has even been applied to interactions between groups. The topic of this monograph, however, concerns the interaction of an individual within a group. But the "group" herein is not just any group. It does not include political associations, institutions, or other sodalities. The common feature of the individual-group interaction that is the present topic requires that members of the group reside in close proximity. The size of the group can therefore vary from an extended family to larger kinships such as a tribe and to a city. Finally, the focus is on primitive groups and the earliest *de novo* appearance of cities in primary civilizations, for the opening question is, did cities originate or survive because of a psychological orientation of humans as "social animals" to reside in close proximity to, or have a need to be part of, an assemblage of many other humans. The answer to this question will be shown to be "No" but that the aversion to larger groupings was overcome in several instances by intelligent self-interest.

It has been the conclusion of *The Natural State of Medical Practice* that, as reflected in the course of civilizations, humans best display their ingenuity when they are free and their capacity for progress when they collaborate in autonomous groups to solve a problem. This was supported by evidence surrounding the evolution of medical practice during early urbanization in several ancient civilizations.

Some have proposed that early urbanization was a consequence of regional population growth, a popular theory implying that cities from the beginning were both desirable and inevitable consequences of increasing population density.[3] The mainstay

---

[1] Aristotle is credited with this phrase, and from his description he seems to be praising citizenship in established Greek city-states (Aristotle, *Politics*, Bk 1, 1253a). The Greek phrase is ὁ ἄνθρωπος φύσει πολιτικὸν ζῷον, in which the literal interpretation implies a need or desire for the responsibility of citizenship in a State. This indicates he was not referring to cities or States in general but in a State where the individual retained political significance.

[2] See the brief review by Simon N. Young, *The Neurobiology of Human Social Behavior: An Important but Neglected Topic*, in *J. Psychiatry Neurosci.*, 33:391-392, 2008.

[3] See publications of Dr. Paul Bairoch, including *Cities and Economic Development: From the Dawn of History to the Present*, English translation, Chicago, 1988. It was Aristotle, of course, who,

for that theory of urbanization was agriculture, for, with the availability of an adequate food supply being the dominant factor, the greater the food supply the greater could be the local population and population density. An adequate supply of food and water therefore was the permissive factor that allowed regional populations to fulfill a natural desire to congregate, something not possible for hunter-gatherers.[4]

An alternative explanation was put forth by Dr. Gordon Childe who considered cities born and bred for commerce. In other words, it was food *surplus* for export rather than food *sufficient* for local population growth that was the key to urbanization. This is a major distinction. In food surplus there might not have been cities were it not for commerce, whereas for food sufficiency humans were just waiting, figuratively speaking, for the opportunity to reside communally with fellow humans.

But if people were so pleased to intermingle then there should have been a city develop just outside Eden's gate, perhaps like Cain's Enoch, that would have enlarged as agriculture prospered until a maximum supportable size was obtained, at which time more distant cities would have emerged. Based on modern scientific theory of human origins, therefore, Africa should have been promptly populated with cities, the other continents laggards.

While Adam and Eve were not hunter-gatherers on leaving Eden, instead pursuing sedentism, evidence indicates it was in small groups that people emigrated from central Africa to populate most of the globe, and there is not a single early ancient city from those earliest days to show for it. This suggests that ideas leading to expanded communal living either did not occur to early people or that they considered that possibility but then rejected it. Assuming we are neither more nor less intelligent that our ancient *Homo sapiens* ancestors, it is reasonable to conclude the latter.

There are, of course, important geological and geographical considerations. One is growing season. Thus, nomadism was abandoned first in more temperate, cooler, regions; the growing season was longer in warmer climes and thus better supported continuation of an itinerant existence.[5] This is an interesting observation in that it suggests any change from a nomadic to a settled lifestyle was the product of geological and meteorological conditions rather than being a lifestyle preference for sedentism, although another possible reason is safety from dangers of the environment or from other humans.

It remains to be explained, however, why it took so many years for the first "cities" to appear following regression of the Quaternary Ice Age. Temporary Mesolithic (20,000-8,000 years ago) settlements have been discovered around the world, suggesting sufficient humans existed regionally during the Ice Age to form sizeable communities but did not. Glaciers had significantly receded 15,000 years ago, yet it took several thousand

---

in his *Politics*, viewed the State as a natural consequence of the desire of humans to associate and live a good life above bare necessity. *The Natural State of Medical Practice*, however, considers the city's "good life" to be the unintended consequence of the original desire of humans to leave the tribal kinship, involvement in commercial ventures being their "escape from egalitarianism" rather than a "flight to pleasure."

[4] Farming requires greater effort than nomadic existence and recent estimates suggest about five acres of land are needed per person for sustenance. There also are problems with soil deterioration and climate changes. Hunter-gatherer groups on the other hand might need two hundred acres or more of territory per person for subsistence. Thus, it has been proposed that population shifts between sedentarism and nomadism and the formation of towns can be explained by the territory needed to provide adequate caloric intake for a given population.

[5] Max Weber, *The City*, in chap. 1, The Nature of the City, Free Press paperback, Glencoe, 1986.

years for a few small and organized settlements to be established, most still being associated with rock shelters and usually occupied only transiently. Locally concentrated permanent populations exceeding ten thousand did not appear until perhaps 6,000 years ago, and even these were all located in or near Mesopotamia, with its earliest 4th millennium city, Eridu, containing perhaps 4,000 inhabitants. Beyond this region there were rarely permanent villages. All this suggests humans were in no hurry to congregate in large communities over the great majority of their existence on Earth even though there would have been knowledge that large settlements could exist or existed.[6] Instead, they generally continued to disperse.

Even when ancient population centers came into existence there was no rush to enlarge them. The population and the accommodations of Catalhoyuk in the 8th millennium remained stable at 8-10,000 for about a thousand years and then disappeared. The early population of Jericho in 9400 BC contain an estimated seventy dwellings. Two thousand years later the population is estimated to have been as low as two hundred persons. Nevali Cori, a settlement in present-day Turkey, comprised some twenty remarkable houses in the 9th millennium, but it was abandoned within a few hundred years. A similar but smaller 9th millennium settlement is at the Gesher archeological site in Israel, and it appears also to have had a similarly brief existence. There are large parts of the world, including vast areas of Siberian and Mongolian plateaus, that have known nothing but nomadic or pastoralist peoples up to the present day. Then there is the modern extreme example of Australian aborigines who, after fifty thousand years of isolation on the Australian continent, have refused to accommodate a single town.[7] There clearly was no pent-up demand for congregating with fellow humans despite glacial regression. There appears to have been little to attract people to either relatively populous or permanent residences if reasonable conditions permitted them to remain separate and nomadic.[8]

To be able to settle permanently in one place (sedentism) required selecting a location with a year-round water supply, a source of game or space for domestication of animals, and protection against uncertainties of weather, geology, and wandering threats, human or otherwise. Sanitation and seemliness associated with permanent human habitation must have been issues. Early centers of sedentism could develop without an agricultural component, but they did not naturally evolve into agricultural towns and cities, and local migratory or nomadic behavior remained a prominent parallel phenomenon. Overall, frequently moving around in separate groups, especially to places known and previously occupied, seems to have been preferable, even though disabled members could be travel liabilities.

But what is meant by "separate?" Is separation a euphemism for autonomy, or does it merely mean a desire to remain in the nomadic, or hunter-gatherer, mode. In choosing nomadic life the band required members who would travel together and remain closely knit to provide for the common welfare. Such groups may go their separate ways, but internally members would be permanently in close contact, with kinship usually being both the common bond of membership and the common authority for obedience. This

---

[6] World population graphics as published by the United States Census Bureau, *Historical Estimates of World Population*, and viewable as of 2021.

[7] See *The Natural State of Medical Practice*, vol. 3, p. 200*ff*.

[8] Perhaps those early populations detected difficult social issues that would be magnified in a city environment. Today's rate of many serious psychiatric diagnoses is considerably higher in cities than in rural environments. See a review of this problem: Gruebner, O., et al., *Cities and Mental Health*, in *Dtsch. Arztebl. Int.*, 114:121-127, Feb. 2017.

was not autonomy. Indeed, as discussed below, the reason for joining in urbanization was not to escape nomadism *per se*, already shown to an acceptable and perhaps even preferred lifestyle, instead being an escape from its egalitarianism.[9]

Agriculture did not change the overall dispersion of the population. Over time the European population increased in part due to immigration, beginning in the 6th millennium, of a farming people via Anatolia and the east. But despite the widespread introduction of farming throughout Europe there are only four possibly permanent settlements dated prior to the 4th millennium, one being Argos in the Peloponnese, dated to *ca.* 5000 BC, a small village. There was a settlement of perhaps a thousand or more individuals near Stonehenge in the British Isles that existed *ca.* 2500 BC, but it was a temporary settlement that lasted for perhaps two or three centuries to support the development of regional henges. Settlements in the British Isles otherwise are inconsequential in size until the 2nd millennium.

Thus, the broad expanse of Europe with an estimated population of ten million by the beginning of the 2nd millennium can be considered virtually devoid of established assemblages of people.[10] In China the same pattern applied but with a twist. Several population centers developed in the 2nd millennium. The early settlement of Taosi of *ca.* 2000 BC is considered the largest center, but the center itself was primarily an elite political habitation with hegemony over a regional population that resided in small surrounding villages. It survived only a few hundred years. The first "urban" site was Erlitou, which reached a population of 11,000 about 1800 BC. It was, like Taosi, a monarchical center. Thus, even within the authoritarian designs of ancient China there was no rush to centralization by the general population, which existed in small satellite villages (a proposed exception to the preceding being Liangchengzhen of the Longshan culture, mentioned below). In the Americas nomadism and semi-nomadism were virtually universal throughout the Archaic Period (8000-1000 BC) and into the Classic Period (500-1200 AD) except for ritual centers. The latter could have commercial functions, generally an appendage in which the common people resided in small peripheral villages.[11]

Thus, despite the immigration from the east that ultimately dominated Europe, the population remained dispersed.[12] Until the subsequent Bronze Age (*ca.* 2000 BC) the British Isles and northern and eastern Europe contained virtually no villages, just hamlets of small clusters of several houses. The same applied to Japan where the largest congregation of the Jomon people, who populated the islands from 14000 BC to as recently as the 1st millennium, was no more than five hundred, almost all other sites being composed of four or five dwellings. In eastern Europe (now the Ukraine and Romanian region) the people of the Cucuteni-Trypillia culture of the 6th-3rd millennia lived for the most part in small hamlets separated from each other by a few miles. But when they did form large "cities" (some with populations of 10,000-30,000) the individual dwellings or small groupings of dwellings were sufficiently separated from their neighbors that each

---

[9] The subtitle of vol. 3 of *The Natural State of Medical Practice* is: *Escape from Egalitarianism*, the theme of the entire volume.

[10] Population estimates available from Statista Research Department, 2007.

[11] Prominent ritual centers, probably with political authority, were found in the Western hemisphere, including Norte Chico (Peru), Cahokia (North America) and San Lorenzo (Mexico), the latter being considered a city that in *ca.* 1000 BC, had a central population of 5500. The first two are discussed in *The Natural State of Medical Practice*, vol. 3, p. 143*f* and p. 151*f*.

[12] *The Natural State of Medical Practice*, vol. 3, p. 246*ff*.

dwelling unit was able to support itself by farming immediately adjacent land. Furthermore, these large population centers did not have commercial centers or monumental structures, thus being more like an amalgam of hamlets.

The seemingly inherent disinclination to crowd together was powerful. Discounting the attraction, usually intermittent, of regional religious or ritual centers, how was it finally overcome? There are two plausible explanations for ancient urbanization. One, more fully treated in *The Natural State of Medical Practice*, provides evidence that commercialization, beginning at the village level and then expanding as local commerce increased, provided an avenue for escape from the egalitarian ethos of the clan or tribe. In this instance the local population involved in commercial ventures increased because people *desired to join* in urbanization.

The other explanation is a need for defense against some external force or threat. In this situation the people felt they had *no choice but to join*, as it was but logical to seek safety in numbers. And this is what was usually done. As a result, groups were larger and regimentation extensive. Bronze Age and Iron Age Hill Forts in the British Isles and throughout Europe are examples of defensive settlements, and few of these became prospering towns or cities. They quartered perhaps a few hundred people, whereas most of the population lived in small and scattered hamlets of about fifty persons. This is the situation that persisted down to within a few centuries BCE when later cultures developed larger defensive settlements such as the *oppida* of the Celts.

In considering the two options cited in the preceding paragraph, the primary civilizations of ancient Sumer, Egypt, India and China began as commercially active settlements, although the Longshan culture cities of ancient China have limited circumstantial evidence to support this claim. But from this we can propose that it was commercialization that led to early urbanization and that its initial success prompted others to join in urban life as a matter of free choice. The result was the city-states of Uruk (Mesopotamia)with an estimated population of 40,000 by 3100 BC, Hierakonpolis (Egypt) with an estimated 10,000 population about 3200 BC, (Mohenjo-Daro India) with an estimated population of 40,000 in 2500 BC, and Liangchengzhen (China) with a population of 50,000 also about 2500 BC.

Considering all the evidence, the conclusion seems inescapable. Humans do not prefer close and integrated contact with other humans if this involves restrictions on their freedom.[13] They are "social" only to a point. In their close-to-natural state in Europe they preferred to live in small consanguineous, or family, groupings near others but not so near that they could easily be pestered, threatened or caught up in the troubles of others. This would have allowed them to visit, befriend and assist others according to family priorities. When Roman Legions threatened they were able to come together and rally thousands of warriors and their families. And since there is no reason to think that we are any smarter or kinder than humans of thirty thousand years ago, the same pattern of thinking is with us today. Thus, cities are an aberrancy, which is not to say whether they are good or bad. In fact, it can be considered that modern cities, despite their countless regulations and social threats, contain some unintended good above and beyond commercial convenience. That good can be considered a consequence of spontaneous order, defined as "order which emerges as a result of the voluntary activities of individuals but is neither a product of the execution of human design nor a creation of government."

---

[13] Parenthetically, it is assumed that leaders of bands and heads of households that determined the course and placement of their respective groups were men, and it is further assumed that women agreed with those decisions. This, however, merits further study. And see footnote reference (15).

The flourishing of the arts and institutions in cities, therefore, has been an unintended product of commerce-induced population aggregation. But it does not escape our attention that a great number of people employed in a modern, safe, and intellectually exciting city prefer to reside outside it.

Does all this relate to natural law which, as explained in Excursus 6, is based on ethical laws that require that we not disrupt the lives of others? We are to respect the right of others to live free; "live and let live." What better way to do this than to live a bit apart from others, thus avoiding uninvited intrusions and making collective action difficult. That this was thought to be the preferred and effective plan of habitation is suggested in the broad application of this plan over vast regions encompassing a variety of cultures for thousands of years. If safety and sufficiency permitted, people lived in small groups where, as pointed out in modern studies of group psychology, there is a greater opportunity for expression of personal opinion.[14] It was only when population continued to increase that circumstances prevailed that increased the likelihood of transgression and violence, thus leading to tribal organization and other defensive arrangements such as Hill Forts and walled enclaves.[15]

On the other hand, the social distancing of small groups, whether by circumstance or by preference, interfered with the opportunity for individuals to share their ingenuity, the basis of human progress.[16] By limiting that interaction Neolithic populations were guaranteed not to prosper or progress. It required a sizeable and stable concentration of people to initiate and sustain progress. What better way to proceed along this path than to embrace a positive incentive for people to congregate and work together. That incentive was a mutually beneficial commercial enterprise. The remuneration for commercial success was not physical victory over another people, instead being a better lifestyle for its members than that existing in kinships. In contrast, Hill Forts or their equivalent were enforced crowding with motivation being safety in numbers. Remuneration was survival, not progress. Freedom was exchanged for security. In contrast, in escaping from the repressive kinship of the tribe the security of social bonding was exchanged for a degree of intellectual freedom.[17]

---

[14] For a comprehensive review of the significance of smaller group size see *Communication in the Real World: An Introduction to Communication Studies*, chapter 13 – Small Group Communication, 2013. This is available from the University of Minnesota Libraries under a Creative Commons Attribution-NonCommercial-ShareAlike 4.0 International License.

[15] Prof. T. W. Luke, in *Social Theory and Modernity* (Newbury Park (CA), 1990) considers this an aberrant response, primarily by males, to "social artifice" associated with crowding (p. 107).

[16] The critical role of the "group" to progress, as opposed to the "individual," is maintained throughout the three volumes of *The Natural State of Medical Practice* and can be summarized as "two heads are better than one."

[17] The definition of kinship, originally based on the concept of kin and representing a common ancestry, has become so diffuse that it is now almost meaningless. Historically, however, it is the ancestral relation, whether consanguineal or affinal, that has guided the major part of humanity over millennia with its rights, responsibilities, loyalties, and protections. But in a democracy where the individual is the source of power and the focus of rights and protections, there is an inherent rejection of a formal kinship, especially in the field of politics. It is for this reason that "social kinships," such as a labor union, a religious faction, a single political party or any type of traditional kinship cannot be allowed to contend for control of our government. Our guarantor in America is our Constitution. Were this not the case, tribal conflict would destroy the political stability of the nation unless a totalitarian government towered overall. Such is the case with China, which for thousands of years has known only kinship-based monarchical or totalitarian rule, and the individual

Viewed in this way, the social environment that permitted progress also permitted personal benefits to benefit others. The concentration of people was no longer a potentially bad thing where proximity bred temptation. Instead, self-interest recognized that peaceful collaboration made it preferable to reside in closer quarters because self-betterment made compromise not only possible but desirable. The importance of compromise is briefly discussed in the opening pages of *The Natural State of Medical Practice*.[18] But it was these interactions of people pursuing self-betterment that would lead to progress, with the accumulation of new medical knowledge that would result from the appearance of a small network of medical practitioners being but one example.

It is reasonable, therefore, to view progress, attributable to a collaboration of persons in which each was working for self-betterment, as an example of spontaneous order, an unintended but beneficial consequence of being in close contact and avoiding violations of natural law (*e.g.*, killing or robbing) in their interactions with each other. And spontaneous order can be viewed as a corollary of natural law.[19] Thus, peaceful dispersion of early human migration and small settlements around the globe avoided higher levels of social repression. When larger and more impersonal kinships developed, peaceful commercial interactions of local assemblages of people (in towns and cities) became attractive, limited social regulation was bearable, and these interactions were the source of human progress. This is not to say that those populations consciously recognized how conducive their choices were with the ethics of natural law.

As for our own time, Western progress also emerged when released from a kinship, this time an embattled pan-European doctrinal kinship embedded into a feudal system. Although no peaceful interlude for collaboration equivalent to a settlement hierarchy ensued, protection provided by a number of northern European principalities and dukedoms permitted initial European steps in religious and later entrepreneurial self-interest. That entrepreneurial initiative has so far survived the political gambits of authoritarianism in the West.

It seems that governments are incapable of refraining from appropriating the products or means resulting from personal attempts at self-betterment for their own purposes, sometimes claiming they are doing so in the best interests of the unprivileged. This is probably the same argument made by an early Pharaoh who might have said to local medical practitioners, "Come join with us and we will make you priests and offer you excellent remuneration, perpetual public acclaim, a temple to live in and access to all the people of the land." Stability was then chosen over personal freedom, and the consequences were terrible.[20]

To summarize the preceding, commercial success invited collaborative efforts that led to population centers and a period of freedom of choice during the settlement hierarchy stage of early urbanization. There was an opportunity to compromise with neighbors on matters of self-interest, provide previously unavailable goods and services, and thereby peaceably improve one's life. That collaboration was possible because compromises necessary for living in close proximity with others were considered a fair

---

remains, except for the present brief toleration of superficial capitalistic freedoms, a mere cipher dependent on government whims.

[18] See *The Natural State of Medical Practice*, vol. 1, pp. 29, 539*f*, 214.

[19] See *The Natural State of Medical Practice*, vol. 3, pp. 273*ff*. Also: Skoble, A. J., *Natural Law and Spontaneous Order in the Work of Gary Chartier*, in *Studies in Emergent Order*, 7:307-313, 2014.

[20] See *The Natural State of Medical Practice*, vol. 1, pp. 71*ff*.

exchange for the benefits derived from commercial ventures. Common needs were met with cooperation, not obstruction. Personal decisions were no longer within the domain of kinships that had denied their members freedom to pursue self-interest since the earliest societies.

What is the lesson to be learned? Dispersion and modest separation in small (usually family) units in ancient times suggest a lifestyle especially compatible with ethical orientation of natural law, a way to avoid transgression on the rights of others and a way to avoid restrictions (positive laws) imposed by larger kinships. By stating it is compatible with or sympathetic to does not imply it was purposeful, and Excursus 4 has made the extraordinary proposal that virtue and progress can exist even in the absence of motive if consistent with natural law.

But the larger the kinship, the greater its power and ability to protect its own. It does so by appropriating the time, effort, and fidelity of its individual members to benefit the kinship as a whole, and, as a kinship grows from an extended family to a clan and to a tribe, likelihood becomes certainty that a chief will emerge and distribute kinship rewards to personal advantage; a primordial politician is born.

Today the government is steadily being given, or is appropriating, more and more authority in directing our personal decisions by declaring it to be in our best interest. It is usurping the role of natural law as it becomes our "chief" and redefines our nation based on social kinships instead of a nation of distinct individuals with personal responsibilities and rights. In doing so, all the failings of the kinship associated with tribalism and tribal rivalries are being evoked as intrusion into our lives is justified by government-defined ethics rather than by natural law ethics. This is because a kinship is, at its core, a defensive unit rather than a progressive unit, a protection against outside threats, and a social Hill Fort appropriate for a pagan and authoritarian world of conflict rather than an opportunity for free individuals to collaborate and compromise in a way that ultimately benefits everyone and leads to progress. Thankfully, a few people from ancient populations left their tribes to join in commercial urbanization, of which we are the beneficiaries. Sadly, in contrast to the clan or tribe, from a government kinship there is no way out. While things may turn out satisfactorily for leaders of the winning tribe, this will not end well for the rest for us. The nation will be easy prey for the authoritarian and the common man and woman will lose again.[21] Would that it were possible for us to safely disperse from our crowded cities, yet retain social safeguards, essential services and our preferred autonomous affiliations.

---

[21] And once again reference is made to the abridgement of *The Natural State of Medical Practice* that is entitled *Medical Science and the Common Man and Woman: A History*, published by Xulon Press in 2020. An eBook version became available in January 2021.

EXCURSUS 8

This excursus reviews human progress as a consequence of liberty of the unprivileged, or common citizenry, and integrates the ancient Hebraic ethos into that sequence. Most religions do not weigh liberty of the individual as a doctrinal element and have not been associated with secular progress. In contrast, the Judeo-Christian religion from the beginning has, in recognizing all people as descendants of God's original creation and therefore of equal importance to our Creator, retained an egalitarian sympathy for human liberty. There were several transient expressions of civil liberty resulting in medical progress in the ancient world. But it was only with the Reformation that there occurred a transposition of that Judaic egalitarian sympathy to governance in the West, the result being two-and-a-half centuries of human progress that have immeasurably improved the lives of billions around the world. This is the first time in human history that civil liberty, the offspring of the ancient Hebrew acknowledgement of the equal status of every individual before God, has been purposely sanctioned and ultimately codified within a civilization, and its astounding success argues it should become both permanent and global.

HUMAN LIBERTY AND THE JUDEO-CHRISTIAN ETHOS

Introduction

In recounting the course of medical practice over the ages as presented in *The Natural State of Medical Practice*, historical aspects of the Judeo-Christian religion unexpectedly revealed themselves, sometimes profoundly.[1] Perhaps this was merely by chance, for the original purpose of examining human history for a natural state of medical practice was to seek pragmatic approaches to contemporary problems negatively affecting the profession of medicine. Still, one must wonder at the similarity in ethical basis of the Judeo-Christian religion and what enabled Western progress. Most religions do not weigh liberty of the individual as a foundational precept and central value. But it is concluded here that Judeo-Christian values are largely responsible for the freedoms which led to the rapid progress enjoyed by Western civilization over the past three centuries.

Using medical practice as a gauge of human progress, three historical periods were identified in which initiation of medical progress could be identified objectively or circumstantially: (1) third millennium early urbanization in Sumer, Egypt, India and China, (2) 5th C BC Greece, and (3) the modern West beginning in the 18th C. A degree of civil liberty is proposed to have existed in each period, with, taking them in order, the first appearing during the interlude in urbanization between leaving the kinship of the tribe and the beginning of authoritarian city-state rule, the second during the interlude between leaving the kinship of the Greek phratry and before the Athenian misdirection of political liberty, and the third following a revolt against a pan-European super-kinship and the codification of civil liberty triggered by the Reformation, a process still under way. The latter can be considered a social culmination of the ancient Hebrew ethos of the importance of the individual before God as expressed in the Pentateuch and its mature Judeo-Christian expression.

---

[1] I am aware of the scholarly and less than scholarly criticism of the term "Judeo-Christian religion" and prefer to ignore that unhelpful debate.

Free Will[2]

Any discussion of liberty must first ask if humans have free will. There has been divided opinion among the world's four great religions, to which over 80 percent of the global population is inclined:

1. Buddhism traditionally does not approach the subject of free will, and this seems consistent with the Buddhist concept of *anatman* in which there is the notion that belief in "self" causes suffering.[3] Recent interest in Buddhism and free will has brought forth controversial opinions on the matter, but, philosophical manipulation being inconsistent, the traditional (for 2500 years) Buddhist view of free will concludes Buddhist ethics and existence proceed apart from our definition of free will as a consequence of human reason.

2. Ancient Hinduism likewise was not receptive to the idea of cognitive free will, although in the 13th C the subject was broached by a "new" school of thought (*Dvaita*) that has been described as "more realistic." But the writings of a Hindu scholar provide an opinion from a century ago stating that Hinduism and free will are incompatible.[4] To avoid philosophical argument, the ancient and traditional view of a dissociation between the Hindu religion and free will is herein assumed.

3. In ancient Islam the concept of free will seems to be explicitly denied. The Quran (57:22) states, in the translation of Dr. Abdul Haleem, "No misfortune can happen, either in the earth or in yourselves, that was not set down in writing before We brought it into being – that is easy for God – so you need not grieve for what you miss or gloat over what you gain." And yet there are freedoms, for Quran states there is to be no compulsion in the practice of any religion. Also, (1) the stigma of not proceeding as ordained by the Quran implies that a person has a choice in the matter, and (2) the distinction between the absolute obedience of Angels and the ability of humans to choose is acknowledged (Quran 2:30). It is also claimed that, as man is God's deputy on earth, he has marginal autonomy. There is modern discourse on the subject.[5] For present purposes it is understood that, while man has freedom to act, the outcome is predetermined.

---

[2] The concept of free will can, in the complex realm of philosophy, be an insurmountable roadblock to understanding. Any preconditioned thinking can be interpreted as the absence of free will. Martin Luther did not consider mankind to have free will because Satan was able to affect one's choice. The use herein is that of Merriam-Webster's "voluntary choice or decision" (Merriam-Webster.com Dictionary).

[3] Repetti, Riccardo – What Do Buddhists Think about Free Will? in *A Mirror Is for Reflection: Understanding Buddhist Ethics*, J. H. Davis, ed., Oxford, 2017.

[4] The great scholar is Swami Vivekananda (1863-1902), who wrote: "Therefore we see at once that there cannot be any such thing as free-will; the very words are a contradiction, because will is what we know, and everything that we know is within our universe, and everything within our universe is moulded by conditions of time, space and causality. Everything that we know, or can possibly know, must be subject to causation, and that which obeys the law of causation cannot be free." *The Complete Works of Swami Vivekananda*, vol. 1, Karma-Yoga, Calcutta, 1907, pp. 95-96.

[5] See: M. S. Uddin, *Far Beyond My Comprehension*, revised edition, CreateSpace, Nov. 2015, original publication by Peace Publication, Sylhet, Bangladesh, and W. Zakaria, *Qadar in Classical and Modern Islamic Discourses: Commending a Futuristic Perspective*, in *International J. of Islamic Thought*, 7:39-48, 2015.

4. Judaism and Christianity for the most part acknowledge the existence of free will, with both free will and natural law in evidence in *Deuteronomy* 30 and championed by Thomas Aquinas (1225-1274), although uncontrollable extraneous factors may affect one's ability to choose wisely.

But, in acknowledging the existence of free will, why was the question asked in the first place? Free will is not synonymous with freedom. The latter is a product of the society in which an individual finds himself, whereas the former, free will, is the ability to consciously make choices. It follows that, for practical purposes, even though a society may restrict an individual's choices, to consciously make a choice is not restricted. It can be concluded that while free will as a philosophical issue may provide an estimate of the significance of the individual in a society, it is irrelevant to day-to-day functioning within that society. The issue instead is *civil liberty*, defined as "freedom from arbitrary governmental interference by denial of governmental power." [6] The status of civil liberty in selected societies/civilizations can now be briefly reviewed.

Civil liberty chronologically considered

1. Four ancient civilizations, 3000-2000 BC

Based on extant medical writings it was proposed that effective medical associations existed in the primary civilizations of Sumer, Egypt, India and China, the respective dates for collection of clinical material proposed as approximately 3000 BC, 3000 BC, 2000 BC and 2500 BC. [7] This was attributed to the spontaneous association of nascent practitioners as the enlarging urban population gradually realized pooled efforts could provide superior specialized services such as medical care, previously a tribal impossibility. Collegial networks in early cities of the four civilizations became possible because (1) there was no authoritarian mandate or social pressure from an egalitarian tribal kinship that might inhibit them, and (2) centralization of political power in early urbanization had not yet developed capable of distorting them. Such a permissive interlude in the social milieu of early urbanization is consistent with an evolving "settlement hierarchy" phase of urbanization in primary cities. [8] The ability to freely associate to further self-interest by providing specialized services that must have accompanied those early medical observations had no doctrinal or communal support, for

---

[6] Political liberty in members of society is defined as being "invested with the right to share effectually in framing and conducting the government under which they are politically organized." Definitions from *Merriam-Webster.com Dictionary*.

[7] The medical writings include: *Treatise of Medical Diagnosis and Prognosis* (Sumer), *Papyrus Ebers* and the Smith papyrus (Egypt), the *Charaka Samhita* (India), and *Huang Ti Nei Ching Su Wen* (China). *The Natural State of Medical Practice*, vol. 1, presents arguments in support of the dates.

[8] *The Natural State of Medical Practice*, vol. 1, chapters 2-5, and vol. 3, chapters 3-6. The early cities of interest were Uruk (Sumer), Hierakonpolis (Egypt), Mohenjo-Daro (India), and Liangchengzhen (China). Each can be considered a city-state. The definition of settlement hierarchy is: "The mechanism proposed as the natural way intergroup adjustments take place as an enlarging population center that has had no prior experience with a leadership hierarchy becomes more complex and must deal with new goods and services needed by the evolving society."

there had been no prior experience with medical professionals and the concept of progress had yet to be recognized.

The proposed dates for the primary urbanizations of the four civilizations far precede the onset of the Mosaic era (ca. 1350 BC), thus precluding any association with Hebraic religion. They also precede Buddhism, Hinduism, Islam and Zoroastrianism.[9]

2. Ancient Hebrews, 1300 BC

As portrayed in the frontispiece of volume 3 of *The Natural State of Medical Practice*, Adam and Eve and the fruit of the Tree of Knowledge of Good and Evil can be metaphorically interpreted as an intrusion into the realm of the Divine in judging good and evil. It can be seen as an attempt by human agents to judge good and evil using their own (arbitrary, subjective) discernment. If effected, the strongest among us would hold that power. The problems associated with human judgment of right and wrong were thus identified in the Pentateuch of the Israelites. And, as that intrusion in Eden indicates, mankind had the freedom to choose (wrongly, in this case). Thus, an acknowledgement of free will can be considered to have been a component of the Hebrew religion by the time of its oral transmission through Moses *ca.* 1300 BC.[10] The escape of Hebrews from Egyptian slavery under Moses has also been used as proof of the importance of freedom to Hebrew society. But humans have been escaping from enslavement by other humans since the beginning of our species, and so it cannot be used as an argument implying that freedom has any particular ethnic affiliation. On the other hand, the Mosaic escape and the resulting Decalogue have been used as proofs of the universal importance of freedom of all individuals, specifically including the enslaved.

It is preferable to limit the discussion of freedom to historic times where there is objective documentation indicating the contemplation or implementation of the concept of freedom, particularly freedom of the individual. Rabbi Robert Gordis expressed a modest but constructive exception to this suggestion in his description of nomadic pre-exile Israelites. Noting that the tribal "*edah*" was a community-wide assembly of men who debated issues pertinent to their respective clans, he considered the democratic and egalitarian ethos of the nomadic tribe to be a restraint on authoritarian tendencies, an ethos carried forward by later Hebrew prophets and ever since a characteristic of Judaism in that there is no voice that must go unheard. One consequence, of course, is the rarity of unanimity on any issue, but, as Gordis puts it: [11]

> Thus for thirty centuries Jewish tradition and experience has exhibited the basic democratic faith that freedom of the human spirit, in all its manifestations, justifies man's audacious faith that "he is little less than God." The oldest living tradition of the Western world would counsel modern democracy that this freedom is to be guarded jealously and to be limited at most temporarily, and then only under the gravest duress of a clear and present danger. It was as an authentic heir of the Hebraic spirit that John Milton spoke when he declared in

---

[9] A possible exception is Ayurveda, which is proposed as originating from the earlier Vedic writings, primarily the Atharvaveda, which some suggest can be dated as early as 2500-2000 BC. The Vedas would subsequently become the basis of formal Hinduism *ca.* 6th C BC.

[10] The origin of the written Pentateuch is debated.

[11] Robert Gordis, *Judaism: Freedom of Expression and the Right to Knowledge in the Jewish Tradition*, in *Columbia Law Review*, 54:676-698, 1954; https://www.jstor.org/stable/1119712.

his *Areopagitica*: "Let truth and falsehood grapple; who ever knew truth put to the worse in a free and open encounter."

It can be concluded that Israelites, as expressed through their true Prophets and Judges, were able to confront and manage disagreements on civil issues often of a religious or doctrinal nature. [12] That this appreciation of civil liberty was retained through many tribulations despite a tribal kinship environment can be attributed to codification during Mosaic times of a Divine covenant, the Decalogue, thereby avoiding the dampening effect of the social egalitarianism in kinships that typically inhibits expressions of individualism.

3.   Ancient Greece, 500 BC

The changes in ancient Greek religious practices have been chronologically compared to the initiation of the natural state of medical practice by Hippocratic physicians.[13] Assuming that Hippocratic medicine was developing in the late 6th C BC, it was a time of diminishing authoritarianism, regression of tribalism, and expanding democracy (*e.g.*, Cleisthenes, 570-508 BC, the "father of Athenian democracy"). Zeus and the Olympian pantheon were becoming the focus of religious thought, and there is no regional evidence of Hebrew influence at this time. Sadly, by the advent of Christianity Hippocratic medicine had, except for the residue of its writings, disappeared. What prompted this brief flourish of scientific progress?

Ancient Greece is viewed by many as a template upon which our modern freedoms are erected. While the argument has been made that Hippocratic medicine and democracy were concurrent events and subject to the same initiating forces, the nature of Greek democracy may make that argument inapposite. It has been stated that while Sparta maintained its military prominence by *indoctrination*, Athens maintained its dominance by *motivation*. But its freedoms reflected the ability of each citizen to argue from a range

---

[12] Even in the opening of the *Song of Songs*, which some think was composed by King Solomon *ca.* 900 BC, where the personages are not clearly identified, it has been proposed that the young woman of the piece forgoes the attentions of the king, returning to her true love, a mere shepherd. This has been interpreted as an indication of freedom to act against even the wishes of a king without fear of retribution, and thus the society to which they belonged must have highly regarded the individual. If the *Song of Songs* was, according to tradition, transmitted orally from King Solomon, the dating would be 10th C BC, but the written version may be postexilic (*i.e.*, after 538 BC). Here is my personal interpretation of the first Song, based on a translation from the Greek of Alfred Rahlfs' *Septuaginta* (1935) by the classicist Dr. Jonah Rosenberg, with gender designations as noted at www.biblegateway.com:

> This is a mini-drama that begins with a young woman expressing her love for a young man. But it is clear that she has been brought to the King because of her beauty. The King says so in verse 1.4, using the "royal we," for this verse in Hebrew is singular masculine. The woman then describes herself as dark-skinned as the camel-hair tents of the Qedars, indicating "medium-skinned," although sunlight could have further darkened exposed skin. Then she reveals her love for a shepherd. This upsets the King, who tells her that she seems to be confused despite all his attentions and therefore she should leave and seek the person for whom she really cares, whom he suspects for some unknown reason to be a shepherd. And so, leaving the King behind sitting on his throne, she seeks her true love. With her attractiveness she finds him, upon which he praises her beauty. She abundantly returns the favor.

[13] *The Natural State of Medical Practice*, vol. 1, p. 458*ff.*

of possible actions required for defense of the city-state, not for personal fulfillment.[14] This is one reason why it was considered so important for each and every citizen to be informed about the issues at hand, with penalties for not voting. It was recognized that for an "all hands on deck" approach to be successful in supporting and guiding the city-state it was critical that every citizen be enthusiastic in the process. What better way than to have him invest his personal well-being and fortune in an outcome in which he had a part in determining and purposely chose, freely instead of by dictate. Thus, Athenians had political liberty but not civil liberty. This is not a new interpretation of ancient Greek democracies. Two hundred years ago Benjamin Constant noted the consequences of the Greek experience with a democracy that included no individual rights, although Athens, because of its expansive commercial activity and interests, was a partial exception.[15]

While not to diminish the importance of those Greek freedoms that existed or Greek democracy, they both were directed at preservation of the city-state rather than personal fulfillment, and therefore they are not relevant to the evolution of medical progress through the efforts of Hippocratic physicians. What, then, allowed a few medical practitioners to see personal benefit accrue by forming a collegial network and sharing experiences from which each would benefit and would improve their services? I argue that Hippocratic medicine was a peripheral and parallel event to Greek democracy, an unintended consequence of the absence of interference with what seemed, to a few practitioners, an obviously desirable plan. There was no law or bill of rights to either prevent or to advance their purposes. But the great thing about Greek democracy was that, apart from social pressures, it *did not prevent* a citizen from advancing personal interests. This is in contrast to kinships, whereby all personal effort is, directly or indirectly, for the perceived greater good of the kinship. Peisistratus (ca. 600 – 527 BC) ended the dominance of kinship in the Attic population as he consolidated the Athenian city-state. In many city-states, including those of the Ionic coast and Dodecanese Islands, this element of civil liberty was permitted to *appear*, after which Greek democracies with their political liberties permitted it to *endure*.

It is therefore argued that there was no etiological association between the freedoms of Periclean Greece and the Hebrew recognition of the importance of the individual. Yet that Greek experience provided sufficient freedom for the initiation of progress, however transient. It is preferable to view the Greek medical innovation, as well as that of the previously mentioned four ancient primary civilizations, as evidence that human progress is an intrinsic, and perhaps inevitable, attribute of human liberty even when that liberty is incomplete and transient, and that even if uninvited it will spontaneously appear provided there are no restrictions.[16] But once success is realized, how can it be retained?

---

[14] *The Natural State of Medical Practice*, vol. 3, p. 304.

[15] "As a [Greek] citizen decided peace and war, as a private individual, he was constrained, watched and repressed in all his movements; as a member of the collective body, he interrogated, dismissed, condemned, beggared, exiled, or sentenced to death his magistrates and superiors; as a subject of the collective body he could be deprived of his status, stripped of his privileges, banished, put to death, by the discretionary will of the whole to which he belonged." Benjamin Constant (1767-1830), *The Liberty of the Ancients Compared to That of the Moderns* [De la Liberte des Anciene Comparee a Celle des Modernes], a speech given in Paris, 1819. Constant was of Huguenot descent and received his education in part from the University of Edinburgh.

[16] Although, as noted in *The Natural State of Medical Practice*, vol. 3, p. 224, a sufficiently large and concentrated population, estimated at 10,000, and several other prerequisites are probably obligatory for producing a medical "profession."

4. The Modern West, 18th C

With the decline of Hippocratic medicine there was no medical progress throughout the Dark Ages and into the Renaissance.[17] But the Reformation released a flowering of independent religious thought that spread throughout much of Europe. Initially this restatement of religious freedom and the Hebrew covenant about equality of all people before God was triggered by Martin Luther's response to the hierarchy of the Catholic Church over purchase of indulgences.[18] But Luther also valued the individual conscience: "A Christian man is the most free lord of all, and subject to none... ," referring to authority within a Christian hierarchy. He considered all people to be "priests of equal standing." By reprimanding contemporary canon law, he was, in effect and whether or not he realized it," espousing equal justice before the law.[19] This is key.

There immediately followed reorganization of many churches that acted upon that concept of religious egalitarianism, with the result that some moved to become independent and self-governing. To prevent governmental infringement on religious freedom this same pattern was then posed as appropriate for secular government.

This interpretation led naturally to a shift toward representative government in many regions because the power of the Roman Church was diminished. The latter had functioned as a pan-European super-kinship or "chiefdom" comprising innumerable "tribes" throughout Europe for 1500 years, and, while its priests and monasteries attempted to provide medical care, spiritual comfort and other valued services to a vast and varied population, its own centralized political power increased to the point that the Church controlled the actions or affected the decisions of many monarchical governments.

With the Reformation this power of the Vatican was contained, especially in the north and west of Europe, because greater was the power of local political institutions. This in turn prompted power struggles between hereditary rulers and increasingly active civilian leaders who sometimes violently fought repressive regimes. The Church was no longer an ally on whom the ruling class could depend. Parliaments were enlisted to assist the ruling class. But with time those parliaments assumed more responsibilities previously held by rulers. Gradually individuals were no longer vassals of the crown, now being able to work motivated by a desire for self-betterment rather than the interests of a ruling hierarchy or the hierarchy of the Church. Thus, the 16th and 17th centuries saw a move toward civil liberties and then recognition of natural rights that released the ingenuity, entrepreneurship, and a desire for special services throughout the unprivileged general citizenry. The fruits of this monumental change began to emerge in medical practice in the latter half of the 18th C, not so long ago!

Usually the Renaissance is given credit for triggering the Enlightenment, in part because it was a time of intellectual rediscovery of the great works of ancient authors, the so-called "Renaissance humanism." But *The Natural State of Medical Practice* provides evidence that little of significance to medical progress resulted from the Renaissance. Instead, it proposes that the Reformation and subsequent political reforms saw the unprivileged, or "common," population bring about medical progress independent of both Hippocratic medicine and the Renaissance. If this an acceptable interpretation of history,

---

[17] *The Natural State of Medical Practice*, vol. 1, book 3, chapters 3-5.

[18] *Disputation on the Power and Efficacy of Indulgences*, the Ninety-five Theses of Luther.

[19] For extensive documentation of this aspect of Luther's work see: Joseph Loconte, *God, Locke, and Liberty: The Struggle for Religious Freedom in the West*, Lexington, 2014.

the Enlightenment itself should also be considered a child of the political reforms subsequent to the Reformation rather than an offspring of Renaissance humanism. [20]

The Mosaic Covenant

Of the several Divine covenants made with ancient Hebrews, the Mosaic covenant (*Exodus* 20:2-17) includes the Ten Commandments discussed in Excursus 6. These Commandments have been an important component of Jewish law up to the present day. The five Commandments that compose the ethical laws are relevant here in that they impose restrictions on our intrusion into the lives of others and vice versa. As interpreted herein and briefly put, they powerfully urge the inviolability of human liberty, and it is our uninvited transgressions into the lives of others, either personally or as a group or as a society, that have checked the variegated ingenuity of our species and prevented human progress for thousands of years.

And this is odd, for the essence of the Commandments is expressed in all societies, advanced or primitive, ancient or modern, where it can be considered a manifestation of natural law, *i.e.*, our conscience.[21] It is almost as if humans were created with an endowed ability to rapidly reach a level of achievement in matters that would improve their status on earth (metaphorically, to achieve a secular Eden), although that ability, unable to be fully realized in the actions of a single individual, required that humans voluntarily work together. Furthermore, *The Natural State of Medical Practice* provides evidence in medical practice that only two or three centuries are needed to initiate rapid progress by this means, once certain demographic and economic circumstances prevail. The problem has been the intrusion by individuals or groups or societies that disrupt or forestall our ability to associate freely. The problem has been authoritarianism in both its political and egalitarian guises as it disregards natural law.

The ancient Hebrew tribes were the first to incorporate this Divine Covenant as a doctrinal force. It has been interpreted as an early form of federalism, for, in contrast to kinship, a covenant does not infringe on the intrinsic character of societies, instead providing a common path for their interactions.[22] Nevertheless, the nomadic ways, tribal rivalries, and captivities prevented basic demographic and economic requirements necessary for progress to be achieved. Thus, Hebrew medical practice, unlike pharaonic medicine, escaped being an authoritarian tool, but it was unable to support a professional association that might have led to scientific medicine.[23]

---

[20] See: *The Natural State of Medical Practice*, vol. 1, book 3, chapter 6. Newton's *Principia* (1687) is sometimes credited with triggering the Enlightenment of the 17th and 18th centuries, but most often it is attributed to "Renaissance humanism," a rediscovery of the ancient writings of thinkers from the Greco-Roman world in philosophy, science, and history. The Enlightenment was understood to be Renaissance humanism's modernization that favored objectivity, sovereignty of reason, the concept of progress, and separation of church and state. It is sometimes credited with the political revolutions of the 18th C.

[21] It has even been proposed that the plan of God for His human creation was revealed to the ancient Hebrews because mankind was seemingly unable to obey natural law and thereby benefit from it; He therefore decided to tell it to the Hebrews directly.

[22] For a review of this concept, see: Fischer, K. J., *The Power of the Covenant Idea for Leadership, Reform, and Ethical Behavior*, in *The Journal of Values-Based Leadership*, 10: issue 2, article 13, 2017.

[23] *The Natural State of Medical Practice*, vol. 1, p. 149.

On the other hand, the Hebrew adoption of the Covenant would permit passage of the message of freedom through many generations of Jews and Christians down to the Reformation. At that point it led to a resurgent appreciation of the importance of the individual, first as a fuller expression of that importance within the Judeo-Christian ethos and then increasing in scope to become a political force that would lead Western civilization to global predominance, doing so not by compulsion but by peaceful intellectual message. In that it explains the critical importance to progress of liberty of the unprivileged, the common man and woman, it has announced the good news of democratic reforms and civil liberties that, if uninterrupted, will continue to better the lives of all people.

If free people, however, through fear or personal pique, continue to voluntarily surrender their liberties to government in return for security, it is predicted that the proven authoritarian consequence, an overpowering political class, could lead to loss of all that has been gained. But, as demonstrated in *The Natural State of Medical Practice*, it will be even worse, for the consequences, being gradual, will by deceit proceed to the point of irreversibility and will then fall full force on our youngest generation and its progeny. This may cause some to reconsider *Exodus* 34:7 and view it as prescient, but by then there will be no escape.[24]

---

[24] The benign nature of the Western ethos that has come to predominate in the world is captured in a conversation by an unnamed member of the Chinese Academy of Social Sciences in 2002 with a group of American missionary tourists, as quoted by David Aikman in his 2008 book, *The Delusion of Disbelief.* I have been unable, however, to locate the original documentation of the quotation, although the statement's conclusion finds support in the article by Robert D. Woodberry, *The Missionary Roots of Liberal Democracy*, in *Amer. Polit. Sci. Rev.*, 106:244-274, 2012. The Academy is a think tank associated with the State Council of China and located in Beijing and unlikely to have officially approved of it: "We were asked to look into what accounted for the ... pre-eminence of the West all over the world ... We studied everything we could from the historical, political, economic and cultural perspective. At first, we thought it was because you had more powerful guns than we had. Then we thought it was because you had the best political system. Next we focused on your economic system. But in the past twenty years, we have realized that the heart of your culture is your religion: Christianity. This is why the West has been so powerful. The Christian moral foundation of social and cultural life was what made possible the emergence of capitalism and then the successful transition to democratic politics. We don't have any doubt about this."

EXCURSUS 9

Epidemiological data extracted from the anthropological and archeological literature of early humans and from other hominids as reviewed here are inconsistent with the argument that *Homo sapiens* is a product of evolution on earth.

AFTER EDEN

> *"Therefore the Lord God sent him forth from the garden of Eden, to till the ground from whence he was taken."*
>
> *Genesis* 3:23

Modern life-styles in the West and in culturally similar countries, regions, and cities around the globe reflect a level of convenience, security, and prosperity for so many people over recent generations that, despite the billions who share little of that abundance, it may seem, especially to our younger population, that prosperity has always been with us, was deserved and inevitable, the natural state of things, and will, with the digital age upon us, remain so. A future without limitations or cares, a secular Eden on a global scale, is eagerly anticipated and is impelling ideological political thought, although overt and pending hazards periodically dampen enthusiasm.

One marker that supports faith in such a future is life expectancy. Biblical statements declare 120 years to be the expected duration of life for humans, and over the past two centuries it has risen for the common man and woman from 30-40 years to almost 80 years in many countries.[1] There have always been exceptional persons, exceptional in health or exceptional in luck, who far outlive the average for their societies, but to have so many live for so long and so well is a remarkable fact of modern times. There is no precedent for this. Perhaps this *is* the path to a secular Eden. Pertinent to that path is human progress, and life expectancy can certainly be considered a measure of that progress.

But first is the issue of priority. Should the increase in life expectancy of modern times be attributed to progress, or is progress merely an inevitable consequence of an enlarging population of older, and thereby wiser, members. The wisdom of the patriarch, the sage, old wise men and women, church elders, oral histories, and biblical declarations (Job 12:12 – "Is not wisdom found among the aged? Does not long life bring understanding?") has reportedly been objectively confirmed.[2] Is a society where children usually do not know their grandparents inherently disadvantaged? If so, then most societies since the first man and woman have been so disabled, and this might explain the slow evolution, perhaps for thousands of years, of progress among humankind.

To answer that question, there are two periods that are usually considered to have significantly longer life expectancies: modern times (proven) and the Classical Age of Greece and Rome (unproven). These two eras are credited with great success in human progress, and perhaps a larger mature and experienced population can be shown to explain

---

[1] *Genesis* 6.3. But the conclusion about the 120-year lifespan is not without its critics.

[2] Li, Y., *et al.*, *Compensating Cognitive Capabilities, Economic Decisions, and Aging*, in *Psychology and Aging*, 28:595-613, 2013.

those periods of progress. There are insufficient plebeian data for the Classical Age, but the issue is readily resolved for modern times. *An increase in life expectancy should precede other evidence of progress* if progress is its inevitable consequence rather than a cause. A recent analysis confirms a significant increase in life expectancy in European populations by 1850, first evident in western Europe and then in eastern Europe.[3] When relating increased life expectancy chronologically to new health-related practices, Europe at a baseline in the 1770s did not realize a significant increase in life expectancy until 1900, the latter including a significant decrease in infant mortality.[4] In contrast, medical progress, a wholly Western phenomenon, began in 18th C Europe with notables such as Jenner (smallpox vaccination), Auenbrugger (percussion), and Morgagni (pathology). Laennec with his stethoscope promptly followed (see Excursus 17). This confirms that in Europe, and subsequently in global populations, *progress in medical practice preceded increased life expectancy*.[5]

And so, with our increase in life expectancy as a legitimate gauge of human progress, what has permitted our species to control, at least in part, our destiny in the first place? Such dominance has been declared or is implied as proof of a genetic *tour de force*, survival in the best Darwinian sense, modern man being produced through a rise in posture, stature, and nature from four-legged or knuckle-dragging forebears illustrated so frequently in cartoons. In this postulated triumphant yet inevitable consequence of the blind chance of a Big Bang, there has been produced gradually more upright, taller, and smarter pre-human specimens. Each little development of each of the big and little bones of the shoulder and spine and toes, each millimeter in height, each microgram of thyroid hormone and each point on the Intelligence Quotient have developed slowly by molecular selection in infinitely small gradations and *in coordination with each other* over millions of years, perhaps with infrequent leaps and bounds of "punctuated equilibrium." The effect of these changes is purportedly to improve mankind's chance of survival in life-or-death competition with other earthly life-forms and myriads of environmental threats that would finally lead to an increase in life expectancy countless thousands of years in the future, specifically our 19th and 20th centuries. If all this is true, what a masterstroke of luck that our ancient forebears accommodated such an extraordinarily tedious sequence of genetically evolutionary events for us, and what a misfortune that they knew not what was occurring.

How did this all progress in the first place, or did it? What set the continuum in motion that stealthily led, over fifteen million years, from the two-foot tall, four-legged, forty-pound *Proconsul africanus* to *Homo sapiens*? If the true human species, *Homo sapiens*, has exhibited society-wide a level of intelligence that has been both unchanging for thousands of years and globally similar, how is it that "survival of the fittest" or natural selection theories can explain the following: that as early as there is objective evidence,

[3] Max Roser (2018), "*Life Expectancy.*" Published online at OurWorldInData.org. Retrieved from: 'https://ourworldindata.org/life-expectancy' [Online Resource].

[4] Using this chronological perspective, extraneous rises such as would occur after plague years in earlier centuries can be avoided. As for other demographics, see: Riley, J. C., "Estimates of Regional and Global Life Expectancy 1800-2001" in *Population and Development Review*, 31:537-543, 2005, and Haines, M. R., "The Population of Europe: The Demographic Transition and After" in *The Encyclopedia of European Social History*, Encyclopedia.com, 10 December 2018.

[5] A more detailed explanation is presented in vol. 1, bk.4, of *The Natural State of Medical Practice*. Complexities of demography are great, and just how much benefit can be ascribed to progress in other areas is a matter of debate, but not here.

primarily from osteology and going back to Paleolithic times, human life expectancy is routinely found to be in the range of 30-35 years, a finding that changes little until the last two hundred years.[6]

In a related observation, the infant mortality rate of gorillas in the wild (*i.e.*, mortality in the first three years of life, including stillbirths) varies considerably although 25% may be a reasonable approximation. But a recent textbook states that Paleolithic humans (9000 BC) had only a 50% chance of survival to age 15, and study of a Bronze Age inhumed population from 500 BC Italy revealed that from 33-50% of the interred were under 5 years of age.[7] Such an abbreviated life expectancy and early childhood mortality occurring in a biological body that is thought to permit living to an age well over 100 years does not seem to be a positive indicator of superior survivability, especially as gorillas, chimpanzees, and orangutans have a life expectancy of 35-50 years in the wild and 50->60 years in captivity.[8]

And at Indian Knoll, a permanent prehistoric habitation site in Kentucky that flourished between 3000 and 2000 BC, a recent reanalysis of data has concluded that, of an interred population over centuries numbering 880, only one was deemed over 50 years

---

[6] Angel, L., *Health as a Crucial Factor in the Changes from Hunting to Developed Farming in the Eastern Mediterranean*, in *Paleopathology at the Origins of Agriculture*, Orlando, 1984, M. N. Cohen and G. J. Armelagos, editors, pp. 51-73. This informative paper has been updated in many ways, but the definitions of life expectancy are so varied, vague, or unstated, that it is difficult to group findings from different papers into one statistical base. The listing of approximate longevities (in years) of ancient populations provided by Angel can be used as a starting place for a general statement such as is discussed here: Late Paleolithic (30,000-9,000 BC) – 35.4 (males) and 30.0 (females); Mesolithic (9,000-7,000 BC) – 33.5 (males) and 31.3 (females); Early Neolithic (7,000-5,000 BC) – 33.6 (males) and 29.8 (females); Late Neolithic (5,000-3,000 BC) – 33.1 (males) and 29.8 (females); Early Bronze Age (3,000-2,000 BC) – 33.6 (males) and 29.4 (females); Middle Bronze Age (2,000 BC and for varying periods afterwards) – 36.5 (males) and 31.4 (females); and Early Iron Age (1,150-650 BC) – 39.0 (males) and 30.9 (females). (Note that dating of major divisions of the Stone Age also vary.) Taking a more specific study for comparison, a well-defined population from a Late Neolithic tomb in Spain dated to 3,700 BC had an average age at death for 38 individual skeletal remains as follows: 17 were "subadult" (under 20 years of age) and 21 were "adult" (over 20 years of age). The mean age of the latter group (male and female combined) was 30.5 years (determined from the average of the individual age ranges reported, minus 7 adults in whom an age range was unable to be determined. Violence was not the cause of death, and they "exhibited a moderate number of pathologies." See: Alt, K. W., *et al.*, (2016) *A Community in Life and Death: The Late Neolithic Megalithic Tomb at Alto de Reinoso* (Burgos, Spain), PLoS ONE 11(1): e0146176. Doi: 10. 1371/journal.pone.0146176.

[7] Stockwell, E. G., and Groat, H. T., *World Population: An Introduction to Demography*, New York, 1984, and Tafuri, M., *et al.*, *Diet, Mobility and Resident Patterns in Bronze Age Southern Italy*, in *Accordia Research Papers*, 9:45-56, 2003.

[8] The Center for Great Apes reports the following life expectancy (in years) for gorillas – 40-50 (wild), 50-60 (captive). Type of gorilla not stated. The National Geographic Institute reports 45 years for chimpanzees (wild), type not stated. Other estimates include orangutans as 35-45 years (wild, with maximum observed being 53 for a female and 58 for a male) and baboons as 30-45. Some local reports give significantly shorter survivals than these estimates, but the difference is generally in the range of only 5-10 years. And a study of chimpanzees in the Mahale Mountains (Tanzania) indicate female fecundity greatest between ages 20-35 years. (Nishida, T., et al., *Demography, female life history, and reproductive profiles among the chimpanzees of Mahale*, in *American Journal of Primatology*, 59:99-121, 2003.) In Dr. Dian Fossey's book, *Gorillas in the Mist* (Boston 1983), appendix C, 9 gorillas on whom autopsies were performed that did not die from poachers included one that was between 50-55 and the other between 55-60 years of age.

of age.[9] The Neolithic hunter-gatherers of the Jomon people of Japan had an average age at death of 36 years if those individuals managed to survive to age 15 years; more recent hunter-gatherers of the Japanese Neolithic who survived to age 15 years had an average age at death of 44 years.[10]

Indeed, very premature death in every age category seems to have been unavoidable until the last two centuries. A reasonable conclusion is that survivability of our early ancestors, or even their first appearance, is not the consequence of a preceding period in which gradual expression of a superior fitness was operative generation after generation. If it had been so, those ancient humans might early on have been gradually approaching that 120-year life expectancy as a consequence of their superior attributes and survivability, primarily due to the complexity of their brain, that their ancestors lacked. Instead, the complex brain of *Homo sapiens* seems to have provided no survivability benefit at all. Evidence even suggests that the life expectancy of early Upper Paleolithic man (considered "modern" man) was no greater than that of roughly contemporary Neanderthals.[11] It almost seems as if humans had not been biologically evolving to inhabit a "survival of the fittest" world, instead just being plopped down in the midst of a dangerous world after emerging from some other state in which their development was guided by quite another process, one in which survival was not predicated on confrontation of danger and chaos, one that was perhaps even Eden-like. If evolution of the complexity of the human brain was not a matter assisting in natural selection, one might wonder why it did so happen.

One unanswered question, of course, is, to what use is the elderly population to survival of a society? If the more complex brain resulted from a selective force for propagation of the human species rather than its longevity, there might be a Darwinian explanation for its development. That, however, would require evidence for increased fecundity or some other mechanism for increasing the number of births and their survival into child-bearing years.[12] Notably, among mammalian species there is instead a negative interspecies correlation between brain size and fecundity.[13]

---

[9] Johnston, F. E., and Snow, C. E., *The Reassessment of the Age and Sex of the Indian Knoll Skeletal Population: Demographic and Methodological Aspects*, in *American Journal of Physical Anthropology*, 19:237-244, 1961. Subsequent reassessments have been made regarding techniques, both osteological and statistical, of this unusual population that displayed much evidence of violence, but the rarity of an "elderly" adult in this ancient Native American population, mostly from *ca.* 3000-2000 BC, is obvious. In the United States in 2016, almost 30% of 300,000,000 people were 55 years of age or older, whereas among the approximately eight hundred Archaic period (8000 – 1000 BC) skeletal remains of Indian Knoll only one was classified as over fifty. The 30% in 2016 can be compared to 0.1% at Indian Knoll, a 300-fold difference or, as usually presented in current popular media, a 30,000% increase.

[10] Kaplan, H., *et al., A Theory of Human Life History. Evolution: Diet, Intelligence, and Longevity*, in *Evolutionary Anthropology*, pp. 156-186.

[11] Bocquet-Appel, J., and Degioanni, A., *Neanderthal Demographic Estimates*, in *Current Anthropology*, 54:S202-S213, 2013.

[12] One area that would have contributed more to species survival than a bigger brain is an increase in fecundity, something impossible to quantitate over the ages, in part because risks attendant to bearing children is blamed for the overall shorter life expectancy of women in prehistoric times, especially for the primigravida. This is one reason why fecundity is not more important in the survival of the human species: its mechanism for success decreases the fecund.

[13] For a recent assessment and review see: C. J. Logan, *et al., Endocranial volume is heritable and is associated with longevity and fitness in a wild mammal*, in *Royal Society Open Science*, 2016 Dec; 3(12): 160622. doi: 10.1098/rsos. 160622.

Thus, the finely tuned biological system that each of us is has so many variables that are susceptible to genetic alteration that perhaps they were meant for some other state. What that state might be has always been the grand question. It is in regard to this that it is appropriate to consider Darwin's conclusion on the construction of the human eye in its complexity and fine integration of functions that permit normal sight.[14] His statement was that it seemed absurd to think that such a complex biological system as the human eye could have been the result of a series of selective genetic mutations whereby each genetic change permitted one member of a species to survive where others could not, that survival benefit being the consequence of improved vision or, in most instances, by chance. Nevertheless, he considered his theory of evolution, first expounded in 1859, to be so excellent that he believed it was the truth, despite its element of seeming absurdity. One wonders what Darwin would have to say about this were he to return today and see the true complexity of the eye and vision as far as modern science has been able to ascertain it. That complexity is so incredibly vast and multifaceted, from the simple optics of refraction to the intracellular production of varieties of cells and innumerable species of proteins that make up the eye's tissues and fluids and their individual evolution and regulation, that modern knowledge cannot be mentioned in the same breath with the simple concepts of the mid-19th C of Darwin. And even now we know our knowledge of the entire process of vision to still be at an elementary stage. Were Darwin here today and aware of all that has transpired in modern understanding, perhaps he would revert to his original position.

And think again about mankind's increase in life expectancy that has occurred only over the past 200 years. There is no evidence of a gradual increase in life expectancy over hundreds of millennia to match the gradual or intermittent march posited in cartoons for early hominid to upright man. Prior to the 19th C life expectancy was in the range of 35 years for the average person, even since the beginning of mankind itself, give or take a few years as suggested by the modest increase geographically and chronologically localized to the Hellenistic period (323-31 BC) (see Table).[15] It was no different from the average of 35 years during the European Dark Ages. It is not hyperbole, indeed, it is a fact, to point out that the common man and woman have, since their very beginning, been living in a perpetual Dark Age except for the last three centuries.

---

[14] Darwin, C. A., *On the Origin of Species By Means of Natural Selection*, New York, 1860, p. 167: "To suppose that the eye, with all its inimitable contrivances for adjusting the focus to different distances, for admitting different amounts of light, and for correction of the spherical and chromatic aberration, could have been formed by natural selection, seems, I freely confess, absurd in the highest possible degree." Modern biology has integrated Darwinism within the larger scope of genetics that many feel dispels absurdity, but the point is best debated elsewhere rather than here.

[15] Life expectancy in the Greco-Roman world is uncertain even though accurate ages of some of the elderly are known. Socrates, Sophocles, Plato, Seneca and Archimedes lived to age 71, 90, 77, 93, and 75 years, respectively, but they reflect the life-style of the rich or famous rather than the average worker or mother. Another major unknown is infant and childhood mortality. Phlegon of Tralles in the 2nd C AD wrote *On Long-Lived Persons* in which he claims to have identified seventy individuals in one area of Italy who lived to be older, some much older, than one hundred years, and Pliny also comments on centenarians in 1st C AD Italy, but see T. G. Parkin, *Old Age in the Roman World* (Baltimore, 2003), especially chapter 6, pp. 173-189, for a discrediting of such claims. The Greco-Roman world was vast and varied, and a meaningful single estimate of life expectancy applicable to either Greek or Roman "culture," especially those of the plebeian class, in that period of history is unavailable.

With the exemption of the controlling elites of human society who, like the queen bee, might live longer because they lived off the efforts of the plebeians, mankind from the beginning has provided little evidence for improved survival because of an ongoing genetic selection favoring some mythical "fitness." Fitness for what? Despite his vaunted brain mankind's life expectancy did not exceed that of the gorilla until 200 years ago.[16] Events suggest instead that man first appeared on this planet quite unprepared for the survival of his species.[17] Despite his capacity for brilliance, life has been for most humans very much as Hobbes noted, short and brutish, but not just from man's unsociable disposition, instead being due in part to an inability to cope.

Table: Mean Stature in Feet and Median Life Span in Years of Humans in Prehistory and History[18]

	Mean Stature (ft.)		Median Life Expectancy (yrs.)	
	M	F	M	F
Paleolithic	5.81	5.47	35.4	30.0
Mesolithic	5.66	5.24	33.5	31.3
Early Neolithic	5.57	5.10	33.6	29.8
Late Neolithic	5.29	5.06	33.1	29.2
Bronze/Iron Ages	5.46	5.06	37.2	31.1
Hellenistic	5.64	5.13	41.9	38.0
Medieval	5.56	5.15	37.7	31.1
Baroque	5.65	5.18	33.9	28.5
19th C	5.58	5.17	40.0	38.4
Late 20th C (USA)	5.72	5.36	**71.0**	**78.5**

Increased age, of course, cannot be viewed as evidence favoring natural selection because at some point increased age and its inevitable infirmities impose a burden on society rather than a benefit, and age-related decreases in fertility obviate any genetic mechanism for fecundity that might otherwise apply, although it might be a marker for other features that are beneficial. As for brain size, it has long been known that the brain

[16] Wich, S. A., *et al., Life History of Wild Sumatran Orangutans (Pongo abeleii)*, in *Journal of Human Evolution*, 47:385-398, 2004, reports wild orangutans reaching the age of 58 for males and 53 for females, and for gorillas the "life span" usually given as 35-40 years in the wild and 40-60 in zoos. Hakeem, A., *et al.*, in *Handbook of the Psychology of Aging*, 4th ed., Birren, J. D. and Schaie, K. W., eds., San Diego, 1996, p. 79, states, however, that "Long-term observational data suggest that the maximum life spans for zoo-living and wild primates may be about the same." (Life span is not the same as life expectancy.) The life expectancy of the same species contemporary with ancient civilizations discussed in this book is unknown, but when available data are compared to that of humans shown in the Table, the point is made: parallel branches on the theorized hominid ancestor tree support the conclusion that life expectancy of humans relative to other hominids is no better and may well be inferior.

[17] Unprepared, unless his preparation was not meant primarily for propagation of his species. But if not for that, then for what? This is an intriguing question that may resonate with natural law.

[18] This Table is modified from that used by: Wells, S., in *Pandora's Seed: The Unforeseen Cost of Civilization*, New York, 2010, p. 23. Measurements of stature could reflect nutritional status. As an aside, note that the male:female difference in height today, 4.5 inches, remains consistent with the Table's data covering more than 10,000 years, suggesting the validity of the data.

of modern man is smaller than some of his proposed forebears and related species such as *Homo neanderthalensis*. Maybe the idea that the size of man's brain has produced his modern mastery of the world has actually been associated with a decrease in brain size rather than an increase. The Neanderthals may have been too smart for their own good.

If man's brain and his fecundity were truly associated with a bettering of his status in life, why, given tens of thousands of years of his attempts at bettering and our great expectations and predictions, has his progress been so middling that in the 18th C Alexander Pope acknowledged him "Created half to rise and half to fall; Great Lord of all things, yet a prey to all;... the glory, jest, and riddle of the world."[19] Whatever has propelled humankind to its apogee has not been its prehistory and early history, of this we can be sure. And whatever humankind was capable of doing 10,000 years ago, it is no more capable of doing now.

But a few hundred years ago something happened, some other circumstance intervened that, after millennia of mankind's milling about in self-imposed incarceration, opened the cage, progress was unchained, with the betterment of the mass of mankind finally improving and doing so at a previously unimaginable rate.

In conclusion, what explains this phenomenon, this sudden appearance of longevity? With human history packed with successes in all sorts of ventures, whether building of empires, climbing mountains, winning great battles, building massive monuments, or growing the largest pumpkin, why is it only now that life expectancy clearly exceeds that of man's fellow hominid, the orangutan? As it turns out, there *is* a path to a secular Eden, a path that is now evident. That path, born of the Reformation and parliamentary process and bred by the Judeo-Christian ethos, is characterized by three features: recognition of the importance of the individual, liberty of conscience (*i.e.*, no restrictions on adherence to natural law), and freedom of self-determination (protection of our natural rights). Their mechanism of operation and its importance in human collaboration and progress have been analyzed in some detail,[20] but for time on earth, for appreciating the pleasantness that life can offer, for the personal interactions with others that provide meaning and fulfillment, a long life, perhaps even one of Biblical proportions, might be desired and attainable, unless humanity reverts to its unpleasant default state.[21]

But why has it taken so long for mankind to realize this path, and will it be permitted to continue the journey? That is the question, and circumstances suggest it is best that it be answered soon.

---

[19] From Pope's second epistle of *An Essay on Man* (1734).

[20] Adams, W. H., *The Natural State of Medical Practice*, in three volumes, Maitland (FL), 2019.

[21] It is curious to note, with regard to Eden, that the calculations of F. A. Hassan ("On Mechanisms of Population Growth during the Neolithic" in *Current Anthropology*, 14:535-542, 1973) show that, beginning with a single fertile couple and a population growth rate of 0.1 percent per year, the total world population at the time of Hassan's article would have been reached in 20,000 years. The present annual rate of global population growth is 1.1 percent.

EXCURSUS 10

Epidemiological proofs presented in *The Natural State of Medical Practice* support the Isagorial Theory of Human Progress. They also (1) support core tenets of Objectivist philosophy and (2) support the concept of natural law. Furthermore, the morality of Objectivism is consistent with that of Judeo-Christianity. Despite its refutation of religion or any intellectual discipline based on faith, the limitations of this Objectivist stance are reviewed and a justification for mutual accommodation is presented. For Objectivism it is central to its philosophy that individuals do not transgress on another's life. In Isagorial Theory that principle is acknowledged to be ancient and cosmopolitan (Judeo-Christian) and active today via the human conscience (natural law). But Isagorial Theory does more than identify the evils of transgression on others. It identifies the primary problem, which is not the individual. It is, instead, authoritarian governance by a political elite. When that authoritarianism is blocked, civil liberty will lead to success of the entrepreneurial group and the community as a whole will benefit. Replace authoritarian governance and there will be little need for philosophy-derived correctives.

AFTER PHILOSOPHY: OBJECTIVISM AND ISAGORIAL THEORY OF HUMAN PROGRESS COMPARED

(Note: The assumptions in this excursus will be more readily understood if Excursus 4, 6, and, especially, 8 have been reviewed in advance.)

Introduction

The Isagorial Theory of Human Progress identifies the source of human progress over the ages, and it may be asked why a modern living philosophy like Objectivism would in any way be sufficiently related to justify inclusion in an excursus. The answer is that (1) Objectivism is in some ways identical to Isagorial Theory, and (2) Objectivism has both a popular and a political presence in today's world. Perhaps they can complement each other.

> **Isagorial Theory of Human Progress: A theory ascribing all apolitical advances for the betterment of mankind to autonomous associations pursuing self-betterment in which each member has equal opportunity to speak freely and share ideas about the group's common interest without fear of retribution. Axiomatically it excludes "betterments" that have been stolen, copied, derived by exploitation, or used for subjugation of others.**

Isagorial theory is a factual explanation of human progress, not a philosophy. If found to be correct it could be used as a guide to prevent regression of human progress that is shown in *The Natural State of Medical Practice* to have occurred in all past civilizations.

In contrast, Objectivism is a philosophy and, like other philosophies, is the study of ideas. Its focus is the individual life rather than advocating a course for civilization, although it favors political guarantees regarding individual rights and entrepreneurial capitalism. Any effect of Objectivism on society is found only in the cumulative effect of its adherents. And to the extent that it has a political face the purpose is solely to protect and advance interests of the individual Objectivist.

While writing *The Natural State of Medical Practice* I unexpectedly became aware of similarities between Isagorial Theory, oriented to society, and Objectivism, oriented to the individual. Moreover, and surprisingly, I found the same features are also core tenets of Judeo-Christianity. This excursus describes those shared features.

In exposing this commonality, it is hoped that the three, in intellectual partnership, formal or no, will strengthen the firewall that must protect humanity from the present menacing power and rhetoric of collectivist authoritarian governance and dogma. If protection is not forthcoming, we will lose the source of, and permit the regression of, human progress obtained thus far.

Some definitions used herein

1. Philosophy – the study of ideas about knowledge, truth, the nature and meaning of life, etc. (Merriam-Webster)
2. Objectivism - the concept of man as a heroic being, with his own happiness as the moral purpose of his life (Ayn Rand). A brief dictionary definition of Objectivism, such as "any of various theories asserting the validity of objective phenomena over subjective experience," is too anemic to be useful.[1] On the other hand, philosophy as an intellectual exercise deals with matters not subject to scientific proof because they "cannot be answered by either observation or calculation, by either inductive methods or deductive."[2] Objectivism, from this description and like other philosophies, cannot be objectively supported by facts even though it is supported by "reason" based only on facts; it is objective in the minds of a proponent because that person's reason makes a fact intelligible in distinct way, but determining what is reasonable about a reason is subject to subjectivity.
3. Natural Rights - the right to life, liberty, property and pursuit of happiness, rights considered inherent and universal (*e.g.*, as described in the Declaration of Independence and supported in the Bill of Rights of the Constitution of the United States of America). I find philosophical support for this interpretation in Prof. H. L. A. Hart's concept of "general" rights: if they are capable of choice, "all men equally have the right to be free," they "do not arise out of any special relationship or transaction between men," and "To assert a general right is to claim in relation to some particular action the equal right of all men to be free."[3]
4. Natural Law – A body of unchanging moral principles regarded as a basis for all human conduct (Oxford English Dictionary). It is the unwritten law in every human being whereby conscience guides discernment between good and evil, thereby protecting natural rights of others from us and advising others to do the same for our natural rights. Opinions differ as to its origin.

---

[1] Merriam-Webster, definition (1).

[2] *The Purpose of Philosophy*, found in: Berlin, I., *Concepts and Categories*, 2nd ed., H. Hardy, editor, Princeton University Press, 2013.

[3] Hart, H. L. A., *Are There Any Natural Rights?*, in *The Philosophical Review*, 64:175-191, 1955. Issues related to legal implications of competing "rights" are irrelevant here.

Origin of our political threats

In Excursus 6 the equivalence of natural law (as *per* Thomas Aquinas in his *Summa Theologica*), the ethical laws of the Ten Commandments (*Exodus* 20:2-17), and the Golden Rule (*Matthew* 7:12) is proposed, with their common message being an inviolable statement on human liberty: Do not transgress (contravene) the rights of others. Through these direct and indirect guides we are able to reason good from bad.

But throughout human history it is the centralized political power of authoritarian governance that has defined what constitutes good and evil for its citizenry, its purpose being to ensure hegemony over the individual by the State. In doing so the State has assumed the position of omnipotence, thereby limiting the options of the unprivileged citizenry to abide by natural law and coercing or tempting them to embrace and comply with mandates often inconsistent with natural law. How does all this relate to the philosophy of Objectivism, which is categorically atheistic and would categorically deny this entire excursus?

Objectivist philosophy is the subject of this excursus because of its uncompromising stand, often condemned for its seeming selfishness, for individual liberty. And it is that protection against infringement on the rights of the individual, regardless of whether one considers them bestowed on mankind or not, that is the principal issue in this excursus. This includes not only protection against infringement by other individuals but also against infringement by institutions, including governance, whether it be governance by monarchy, oligarchy or majority.

The issues

Despite the similarity in Objectivism and Isagorial Theory regarding freedom, as a philosophy of life Objectivism is profoundly personal and promotes freedom to unshackle man so as to enable him to lead a moral life guided by his reason. Isagorial Theory, on the other hand, works through society and promotes freedom to unshackle society so as to foster progress and make a civilization civil. This excursus will attempt to show that Isagorial Theory rides shotgun for philosophies opposing authoritarianism in general, but that it is most consistent in the implementation of Objectivism. It is, however, inconsistent with the tendency of Objectivism to avoid any association with religion, defined generally as faith in a god or God but usually directed at Judeo-Christianity. That stance will be shown to be both unnecessary and counterproductive.

Objectivism is a philosophy that, like other philosophies, has been the source of endless discussion, criticism, praise, and sophistic hairsplitting. It is true that Objectivism is a fully developed philosophy, whereas Isagorial Theory is proposed as merely an explanation of the mechanism of human progress. In fact, my studies that led to Isagorial Theory were to determine what could provide medical practice with guidance in the future, not to advocate for a philosophy of life. But it is argued that, without that history of freedom for the unprivileged, the "common" men and women as recognized by the Isagorial Theory of Human Progress, a philosophy of life such as Objectivism could never have come into existence. One reason to compare Objectivism with Isagorial Theory and to promote its co-existence is to maintain aspects of the social environment that permitted Objectivism to appear in the first place and influence mankind for the last seventy-five years in hopes that it will continue to do so.

Objectivism may be fine for the individual, but does it harm or improve the condition of others? If what is good for that individual is good for other people, then it (unintentionally) does good. It could be the good done by the individual Objectivist, or it could be the spread of Objectivism to other individuals that permits them to improve their personal condition. This is an important question because (1) it may ally a valued personal philosophy with our attempts to continue to improve the conditions that surround our daily lives, and (2) Objectivism would acquire an element of scientific objectivity (unequivocal human good; see Excursus 2) that supports the usefulness to others of a philosophy based on human reason that specifically excludes contributing to the benefit of society as a purposeful goal.[4] Let us examine areas of common interest for Isagorial Theory, Objectivism and Judeo-Christianity: morality, natural rights and natural law, Judeo-Christian ethos, faith vs. reason, free will, virtue, and capitalism.

1. Morality:

The following statement of Ayn Rand is at the core of Objectivism:

"… each individual morally must be left free to act on his own judgment – and each individual morally must leave others free to act on theirs." (found in *Ayn Rand's Theory of Rights: The Moral Foundation of a Free Society*, Craig Biddle, 8/20/11. This is a good synopsis of Rand's ideas.)

This statement represents moral absolutism and thus is meant to apply to everyone. Objectivism rejects working for the common good *per se* and, to the extent working for the common good detracts from rational self-interest, would consider such an action immoral, certainly so when coerced. In Isagorial Theory of Human Progress, however, it is shown that acting in rational self-interest (usually via an autonomous group, or koinon [κοινόν]; see *The Natural State of Medical Practice*, vol. 1, p. 168*ff*) is the source of the ideas and impetus that improves not only the condition of the individual having the idea for personal betterment but also the other members of the group, and it may ultimately further the common good, *i.e.*, an "unintended good" or example of "spontaneous order," and not immoral in the eyes of Objectivists.[5] It may be, therefore, that there is no need to distinguish between the morality of self-interest and the common good in a free society. When they move together the ship will right itself regardless of motive. And they will always move together, for entrepreneurial benefits are realized solely via their popular response. The two are thus inextricably associated (See Excursus 4 for more on motive). At the least, Objectivism and Isagorial Theory can be mutual but distinct partners. If this is so, popularization of Objectivism could be an unintended good for society. All of this is not a new idea, for Ayn Rand considered capitalism beneficial for the poor, although that was not its purpose. It is proposed that Objectivism, like the Isagorial Theory of human progress, can be associated with and can promote this approach to the unintended common good, *in effect an intentional unintended good: we know it will produce good; we just don't know what that good will be.* In this setting, Isagorial Theory explains a

---

[4] Cleary, S. C., *Philosophy shrugged: ignoring Ayn Rand won't make her go away*, in the digital magazine *Aeon*, June 22, 2018.
[5] Ayn Rand, in the *Ayn Rand Lexicon* (1986) states that "the common good" is a "meaningless concept."

mechanism that helps clear the path for human progress, and Objectivism arms the individuals that will use that path.

In Objectivism it is not the thought of doing good for society that is the issue. It is, instead, the immorality of infringement on the time and effort of the individual who is striving for self-betterment or the moral weakness of that individual in permitting himself or herself to be involved or exploited in such a misguided effort that is the problem. Of these two categories of missteps, external coercion would be immoral, but one may truly want to help one's friends or neighbors or groups in other countries in trouble, and this is an expression of humaneness. As discussed in *The Natural State of Medical Practice* (see vol. 1, p. 327*ff*), humaneness is a virtue and, while virtue is inversely proportional to the authoritarian rigidity of a society, the free society of Objectivism would value it. Humaneness as a virtue is expressed in the novels and personal life of the pioneer of Objectivism, Ayn Rand. There is no issue here; the "common good" should not be a dirty word in Objectivism and a humane act is virtuous so long as it is not commanded.

Also to be considered is whether Objectivism can be associated with evil. Can it at times be considered immoral? In espousing categorical atheism does it take a metaphorical bite from the fruit of the Tree of Knowledge of Good and Evil and in doing so define good and evil on its own terms? It does not, either functionally or ethically according to the Judeo-Christian tenets as expressed in natural law and the ethical Commandments. This is because the definition of immorality in Objectivism and in Judeo-Christianity is similar. Admittedly Objectivism utterly opposes the Golden Rule's seeming altruism and self-sacrifice. But Objectivism should be judged by the Golden Rule inversion, the "silver" rule. The latter can be stated thus: "Do not do unto others what you would not want them to do to you." (See Excursus 6 for why this is preferable.) To do so is therefore immoral, and this is implied by Ayn Rand in the quotation above. Thus, Objectivism is not a source of evil for society and is in complete sympathy with this core Judeo-Christian tenet, the reason being that it has, through its "reasoning," arrived at the same final product.

As for the immorality of coerced working for the common good and its effects on human progress, that is the consequence of authoritarianism rather than a matter of philosophical incontinence of a society. It is a matter of too much power in too few hands of persons who shouldn't be given power, preventing which is the great virtue of a democracy that disseminates power among the people. The people in China do not lack a desire for freedom, a desire to pursue self-betterment, or competence in creativity and progress. It is the few people holding power and enforcing immoral regulations that are the problem. In other words, rarely is the dilemma of arrested self-interest purely a matter of philosophical immorality or personal choice; it is instead simply a matter of reaction to external authoritarian coercion made possible by centralization of power in the hands of a few, and at times that coercion can be physically brutal. Given freedom to pursue self-betterment, human progress will inevitably occur, will be multifocal, and will disseminate power. The answer to coercion is to stop the coercion. And this is a critical point: it is not necessary to change people's minds. Their minds will rationally change when the coercive force is removed. With the immorality gone, morality will resume its rightful place, as long as no other authoritarian coercion appears and prevents it. Immorality is perpetrated by those who personally interfere with and coercively attempt to direct the lives of others, for they, the transgressors, are the problem, not the perversions of abstract philosophies. In the matter of Germany and WW II, the basic problem was Hitler and the Brownshirts, not Heidegger or national identity. And the freer the society and less the centralization of power, the less of that type of transgression of natural law there will be. But what is natural law in this context?

2. Natural rights and natural law:

The importance to Objectivism of rights that many construe as "natural" was understood by Ayn Rand, but she stated they cannot be justified except by reason and logic:

> "[To] rest one's case on faith means to concede ... that one has no rational arguments to offer ... that there are no rational arguments to support the American system, no justification for freedom, justice, property, individual rights, that these rest on a mystic revelation and can be accepted only on faith – that in reason and logic the enemy is right." (Ayn Rand, *Conservatism: An Obituary*, in *Capitalism: The Unknown Ideal*, New York, 1967, p. 197.)

But natural rights, as considered in the Declaration of Independence, are acknowledged as self-evident (*i.e.*, obvious by means of human reason). In this sense of "reason," and for the purposes of discussion herein, their discovery by reason is similar to that of Objectivism. But some consider rights to life, liberty, and pursuit of happiness as given by God, and thereby natural rights are protected by natural law.

Natural law goes unmentioned in Objectivism. In contrast, centuries, even thousands of years, of reasoning concludes that natural law is inherent and universal and represents our given ability to judge what is good and what is evil, and our natural rights are "goods" that natural law protects. Natural rights say John has a right to life, and natural law therefore says to everyone, it is immoral to take John's life. The latter is a law laid out in our conscience, although a penalty is not specified for disregarding it. It is society that determines the penalty using human reason and man-made ("positive") laws. Actions taken in accordance with natural law are moral and as discussed in the preceding section are considered consistent with Rand's Objectivism morality. (Also see Excursus 3.)

Thus, there would seem to be no quarrel between Objectivism and Judeo-Christianity about the appropriateness of natural law whether reasoned or not. But there is a difference: in Objectivism natural rights and their protection are arrived at by reason to serve the purposes of an individual, whereas the Judeo-Christian view is that while natural rights and natural law do serve the individual, they, being inherent and universal, also serve everyone; *i.e.*, they have a broader domain and *serve to stabilize human society; they are our guide for getting along with one another*. The reasoning and logic of Objectivism merely arrive at what is already universally understood by many to be natural law. It is just that Objectivists would (1) disavow any preexisting purpose, and (2) consider the greater social effects to be irrelevant to their philosophy. The issue is more a matter of editing than composing. In a sense, Objectivism might be viewed as natural law in practice rather than being just another philosophy.

In another difference, in those instances where natural law is obviously being disregarded, Isagorial Theory of Human Progress has shown that the problem is authoritarianism, specifically political and egalitarian. Man-made law or enforced ideologies in those instances have overshadowed recognition of natural law (which is expressed via our conscience). Thus, natural law is expressed to varying degrees according to circumstances surrounding the individual. In Objectivism natural rights and their need for protection are discovered, all or none, by logic and reason of the individual. There is no half-way Objectivist, whereas natural law becomes evident to all via our conscience to the degree that each individual is willing or able to express, and this can be profoundly affected by external political forces. The issue here should be cooperation rather than an inferred competition.

Despite differences, Objectivism as a philosophy and Isagorial Theory as a social mechanism are both staunch advocates of natural rights and natural law, even though natural law is not mentioned in Objectivism because it presumes natural law to be mystical in origin. By facing down Rand's "enemy" in separate battles, personally and comprehensively, Objectivism and the Isagorial Theory of Human Progress would be better off side by side.

And consider the following. Objectivism states that we come to value freedom and our rights on the basis of reason because to be free is natural, *i.e.*, it is moral reality. But no one suddenly comes upon the components of Objectivism already in place. It took years for Ayn Rand to develop her philosophy. It developed as a result of her analysis of her life experiences and scholarship, and its popularity for others is a consequence of the attractiveness of Objectivism as a fully developed philosophy. In contrast, Isagorial Theory views natural law as inherent in everyone in every age regardless of the society, although it is less perceptible when overwhelmed by man-made laws and ideologies. One might therefore consider that it was a stimulus emerging from natural law that lay behind Rand's desire to memorialize her insightful philosophy in writing, even though presumably she would deny it, saying it was instead based on reality; it was "natural." That, of course, is absolutely true. But in either case, when authoritarianism is minimized, functionality of natural law can, via our conscience, be more readily appreciated and implemented, can assist us in protecting our natural rights, and can keep us from interfering with those of others, *i.e.*, it assists us in making "good" decisions as well as being good neighbors.[6] Rand was able to let us know of her new philosophy in our (relatively) free society. She didn't "discover" Objectivism. She considered elements of it in university, "invented" it on coming to a free America, embellished it, and was sufficiently prescient to write it down in a compelling form. It is a reasonable speculation, therefore, to consider Objectivism, in part, as a particularly profound but personal argument for the existence of natural law, one made apparent after she left the world of repressive man-made laws and immoral ideologies of Russia.

3. Judeo-Christianity:

Excursus 8 discusses the Judeo-Christian ethos, its relation to individualism and freedom, and its place in the initiation of human progress that has guided the West, and subsequently the world, since the Reformation. In a teleological sense, it has helped make

---

[6] Why is natural law so readily overshadowed by man-made ("positive") law? Perhaps there is a reason. Is natural law sometimes wrong? I think not and would rather agree with the suggestion that man-made law is our response to some clear and present danger and sometimes is essential for survival. In practice, therefore, it has been sculpted so as to allow us to temporarily appear to supersede natural law because unanticipated needs of mankind and threats of the world inhabited by mankind. Natural law is of a general nature that can be applied to a variety of circumstances by any individual, whereas positive laws are society-specific and meant for specific problems that develop along the way. Natural law is neither mystical nor subjective. It is real and is expressed in all societies (see *The Natural State of Medical Practice*, volume 3, p. 273*ff*).

the world safe for Objectivism. It concludes, arguably, that had not the Reformation occurred the world could still be living in the 15th C.

Individualism and freedom, of course, are the *sine qua non* of Objectivism. But Objectivism the philosophy is a product of the mind of one person in the mid-20th C. The vast leaps in individual wealth and well-being around the world have not resulted from ruminations on the benefits of an Objectivist philosophy. Nevertheless, it certainly could be argued that Objectivism has contributed to the recent Western, and thereby global, progress traceable to the Reformation, if for no other reason than many prominent and successful persons in the West have espoused or admired its message. But the point is, without Western freedoms there would be no such thing as Objectivism. No other culture would have permitted it. It is unexpected, therefore, that there has been expressed no affinity of the one for the other (*i.e.*, Objectivism for Judeo-Christianity).

One explanation for this detachment can be laid to the rigid exemption by Objectivism of anything that smacks of the metaphysical as defined by study of matters outside objective experience, which includes spirituality and faith. And yet, as human progress was begat long before Objectivism and as Objectivism itself exists as a consequence of freedoms traceable to the Reformation, there seems to be no reason for reticence against religion. In fact, there is superficial similarity between Objectivism and Reformation views. In the latter it was sometimes considered a right and responsibility to render oneself prosperous and fit, because to purposely become poor or infirm means one becomes a liability to someone else and cannot be of assistance to anyone should that occasion be necessary. In fact, being self-reliant and prosperous was considered evidence of a blessing from God to the point that religious donations became unpopular. And Judeo-Christianity has no quarrel with a philosophy of individualism and freedom whose popularity is possible because of Judeo-Christian tenets. If Objectivism would but acknowledge there is no moral incompatibility between Judeo-Christianity and science, which there is not (Aristotle and Aquinas have much in agreement on this point), it would move Objectivism to the forefront of the dominant philosophies.

4.   Faith vs. Reason:

Lifelong, most human decisions are based on reason, so a discussion of basic reasoning is unnecessary. Faith is reasoning based on a relative level of confidence of something. It is, therefore, a corollary of reason but is inculcated to varying degrees. And that is their basic distinction; the ability to reason is inherent, but faith in what is reasoned depends on experience and circumstances, and the degree of faith for the most part depends on one's estimate of the risk, or chance, or opportunity, of something being true, and this includes those who, in the presence of honesty, unconditionally accept the opinions of others who base their "faith" on evidence.

Objectivism considers it unnecessary that the world have a cause, and to speculate on the matter is of no consequence and even pernicious. But to say that our universe has always existed or that it popped into being out of nothingness is incomprehensible. Everything we objectively know through our senses had a beginning and a cause. To think otherwise is therefore logically unreasonable. Humans have universally felt a need to hypothesize on the beginning of our world, and to speculate on its cause is a reasonable first step. It is a very basic step because it is an expression of natural curiosity, which is to explore those things which seem inconsistent with prior observations. Thus, we look for a reason. It is not only reasonable; it is natural and even transpecific; curiosity killed the cat. It would be unreasonable to expect or require a person to forego his curiosity about the origin of the universe or our world. In this sense, Objectivism has arbitrarily positioned itself beyond reason.

More in question here is not faith in one's ability to estimate risk in the material world: the strength of a rope, one's ability to jump a crevice, the abscess healing on its own. It is metaphysical faith. Metaphysical faith is sometimes considered at the far end of a spectrum of what might be called wishful thinking, and it is said to contain no objective elements of proof. But metaphysical faiths often claim to have proofs that support the faith. This is natural, for proofs aid understanding and bolster faith by increasing the chance something is true. Samuel Johnson, although a passionate communicant of the Church of England, was said to eagerly seek evidence surrounding reports of miracles. He sought additional proofs despite his faith.

But are not material faith and metaphysical faith the same? Reason and logic are actually insufficient in themselves to serve our best interests unless they embrace faith. Many decisions require faith (in our ability to estimate risk or chance) when they are implemented. Faith in oneself is necessary for many of life's successes. As another example, the Isagorial Theory of Human Progress may be useful, for it is a theory, not a hypothesis, and it is supported by objective proof as presented in *The Natural State of Medical Practice*. While it is indeed a theory, we can have faith in its relevance to society to the extent that its proofs are deemed sound.

It has been stated in Objectivism that "atheism is not a negation, but rather an affirmation of reality, of reason's ability to know it, and of man's ability to create meaning for himself." In such a philosophy everything becomes relative, just as it was for Nietzsche and Sartre. But atheism as a disdain of faith is merely a side-show to Objectivism. It nevertheless needs as much thoughtful consideration as any other doctrine. Varieties of atheism include ethical, psychological, metaphysical, pragmatical, and epistemological.[7] The value of this list by George Hamilton Smith is in its identification of the self-defeating logic those types of atheism present. It conveniently delegitimizes them for us, thereby greatly reducing the number of atheistic arguments that need to be addressed concerning the atheism of Objectivism, and the latter is, simply put, opposition to any form of mysticism. If, however, Judeo-Christianity is found to not be mystical, even in part, then the wall between it and Objectivism may be breached.

To the above point, Judeo-Christian faith abounds in truths. Biblical descriptions are increasingly scientifically verified as modern scientific techniques have made a search for them possible.[8] The case is easily made that one can justify faith in the Bible because it has been proven to be a valid literary source for, and confirmation of, many historical events, predictions and persons, including those relevant to Judeo-Christianity itself. If all the check engine lights are off, we have a fair level of faith that our car will not break down when we drive to the store.

But it can be argued that even if the mysticism argument remains intact, there may be a gate through the wall. Faith (from *fides*: trust or faith, as in *bona fides*, in good faith) is trust, and that trust is based on one's belief on the certainty of something. It is, therefore, a corollary of reason, for it represents a reasoned estimate of the risk, or chance, of something being true, as described earlier. It is argued, however, that faith is that amount of confidence we have in something that is *beyond what is realistic or reasonable*. But determining what degree separates realistic or unrealistic is a function of reason, and it is but natural that there will be varied estimates of that degree. Instead, Objectivism

---

[7] Smith, G., *Atheism & Objectivism*, in *Reason*, Nov., 1973.
[8] Metaxas, E., *Is Atheism Dead?*, Washington, DC, 2021.

objects to any evidence whatsoever of the mystical, the latter defined as "neither apparent to the senses nor obvious to the intelligence."[9] But the Judeo-Christian faith is based on oral and written commentary documenting its early appearance and rise. Assuming several overlapping accounts of aspects of the life of Christ were the basis for the four canonical gospels (admittedly a debated point), Samuel Johnson could state that, given the remoteness of the events, the similarities among the four gospels would represent a level of scientific proof of the accuracy of the New Testament that most science would envy. Judeo-Christianity is not a fairytale first dreamed up by a drugged shaman. Proofs abound that support its historicity. It is only the *degree of reasonableness* in interpretation of those proofs that should be the issue, not a "yes" or "no" on the proposed proofs themselves. And so it is the "degree of reasonableness" that is the gate through the wall. If that gate is kept shut, it will prove the unreasonableness of Objectivism and sadly link it with the illogic of the other forms of atheistic philosophies that will gather dust on the shelves of academics.

I won't mention here the idea of seeing through solid opaque structures in 1894, which would surely have been considered mysticism.[10] But it has been argued by many that life itself is an incontestable miracle that science, despite decades of directed study, is absolutely unable to explain. This is incontestably true. As life clearly exists, it is those who deny it being a miracle of ordered creation that are displaying the greater faith. Objectivism should qualify its delegitimization of the Judeo-Christian faith and remove categorical atheism as an exclusionary philosophical principle because atheism and non-atheism are both faiths.[11]

5. Free will:

In espousing free will, Objectivism joins with Judeo-Christian tenets as laid out in Excursus 8. It also distances itself from other major "religions" that find significant problems with the concept of free will. Zoroastrianism is an exception.

6. Virtue:

Craig Biddle has listed some virtues consistent with Objectivism, including independent thinking, productiveness, justice, honesty, and self-interest.[12] Varying lists of virtues accompany various philosophies. But what are deemed virtues in one circumstance may not be so in another. Loyalty to one's fellow gang members engaged in robberies is not a virtue. And as discussed in *The Natural State of Medical Practice*, virtue is considered impossible in the absence of freedom, and so the above listed virtues, as qualities necessary for adhering to one's philosophy of life, could be altered or redefined to accommodate the State or made impossible in a strictly authoritarian world. In contrast, it was argued in *The Natural State of Medical Practice* that there is one overarching virtue that is a constant in any circumstance and cannot be turned into something monstrous, and that virtue is adherence to natural law (see Excursus 4).

---

[9] Merriam-Webster.com Dictionary; https://www.merriam-webster.com/dictionary/mystical.

[10] In 1895 Wilhelm Roentgen discovered, by a coincidence, "X" rays.

[11] To believe that our universe has always existed or resulted from an arbitrary physical explosion out of nothingness based on proofs in hand requires an enormous leap of faith. At least creation by intelligent design is based on logical reasoning.

[12] The article by Craig Biddle is found at www.TheObjectivistStandard.com, Feb., 2014.

If we take self-betterment as a virtue in a free society, how does it hold up as a virtue in the Isagorial Theory of Human Progress. Adherence to natural law prohibits taking something from others without their consent. It follows that mere existence requires that a person be self-reliant.[13] The degree of subsistence is irrelevant. To live in a humble disheveled hut or in a stately mansion depends on the social orientation, opportunities, abilities and priorities of the individual. In either case, if self-reliance is maintained, that virtue is maintained. All humans, as proposed in *The Natural State of Medical Practice*, will inevitably engage in efforts to progress if not impeded and will usually do so by associating in groups with a common goal of self-betterment. Thus, self-interest is (1) a virtue assumed by natural law and (2) specified as a virtue by Objectivism, and its value is unrelated to individual accomplishment. It is, instead, related to not taking something from others without their consent, *i.e.*, adherence to natural law. The point is that self-interest and personal responsibility, both in Objectivism and in Isagorial Theory, are consistent with natural law as a Judeo-Christian tenet.

For the virtue of "honesty," natural law views prevarication in all its forms as immoral, for by lying to another person we are denying him access to the truth of an issue and thereby interfering with his true understanding of it, and to varying degrees his welfare relies on knowing the truth of the matter. The Objectivist values honesty as adherence to the facts but does not view it as a social duty, instead considering it a negative reflection on the person doing the lying because the "real" message is changed into an "unreal" one and thereby reveals a sacrifice of one's reality, an Objectivist sin. Thus, in both natural law and Objectivism a moral defect lies with the person delivering a lie, although Objectivism carries the etiological blame for the lie further by damning its philosophical irreverence, whereas natural law considers philosophical justification unnecessary: it is bad just because it is something you would not want anyone to do to you.

7. Capitalism:

Both Objectivism and Isagorial Theory fit comfortably with natural law regarding entrepreneurial capitalism. Isagorial Theory optimally functions in a laissez faire capitalist system, and its successes spread throughout a society and reinforce the importance of capitalism. Similarly, Objectivism recognizes capitalism as the only valid socioeconomic system. But in Objectivism capitalism finds its moral justification in serving the individual as it is the individual "capitalist" that benefits from the freedoms of entrepreneurial capitalism. Isagorial Theory also relies on the individual, but its engine usually is a group of individuals acting in self-betterment, and thus it provides a mechanism that benefits each of the individuals in that group. But for both Objectivism and Isagorial Theory the whole idea of an entrepreneurial capitalist system is to more efficiently provide something sought by society at large. Thus, while looking after self-interest, they both are doing what is considered desirable for the community at large, or at least part of the community; they wouldn't be doing it if others in the community didn't want it and were not willing to pay for it. Objectivism is thereby willfully functioning for the common good despite Rand's pronouncement that the common good is "a useless concept." In fact, the greater the resulting common good, the greater would be

---

[13] There is moderation on this point, however, for physical or mental disability and immaturity are circumstances that in a humane world require assistance, and proffered assistance would be desirable and virtuous.

recompence for services or products rendered. Rand, of course, was criticizing "common good" as a goal of such an effort, whereas both Objectivism and the Isagorial Theory support it for its personal benefits, the latter merely being certain that they will appear.

The preceding paragraph, in describing the good for an entire society that might develop from an individual or group's self-betterment capitalistic effort that was unintended or even unimagined at its initiation might be considered an example of "spontaneous order." For a discussion of spontaneous order, see *The Natural State of Medical Practice*, volume 3, pp. 257-258.

The unique usefulness of Isagorial Theory

Isagorial Theory of Human Progress, by defining those elements necessary for progress that have led to a longer and better life and doing so by adhering to natural law, decreases the need to apply a philosophical corrective for the distressing social environment that authoritarianism has caused in the first place. Much philosophical speculation regarding a better world might then be better used on other issues, rather than trying to square the ideal with the real.[14] If Isagorial theory is correct in representing the real world and the threat of centralized political authoritarianism, the more it is implemented the less will be the need for or interest in philosophies that blame our problems on other things, such as capitalism, religion, and lack of will. Freedom would have made those objections irrelevant.

At the present time, Objectivism can be viewed as a defensive philosophy in an authoritarian world. It is a response to authoritarianism and a moral corrective for the individual in an immoral authoritarian society. But the freer the society, the easier it is to adhere to natural law, and the less is the need for a corrective because infringement on individuals would be less common. Individuals will be freer to advance their own interests and thereby would be more restrained in their attempts to transgress the freedoms of others. There would be fewer injustices that require us to impose our own solutions to social problems we think have been created by others. The reason? There would be fewer social problems because everyone would be better off, both physically (because of more prosperity) and psychologically (because of fewer threats). And the simple explanation is this: freedom from infringement on natural rights.

For Objectivism it is central to its philosophy that individuals do not transgress on another's life. In Isagorial Theory that principle is acknowledged to be ancient and

---

[14] Wikipedia lists 416 named philosophies (admittedly some are technical), each one considered significant enough to justify a "search." And as an example of commonality of philosophical thinking, it has been stated that in India "every man is a philosopher." Surely this is so world-wide, from which we can conclude that upward of six billion philosophies exist, each one different and each one an expression of an individual assessment of one's proximate world. So why craft a particular philosophy in such a way that it appeals to a large audience? And if we are content with our personal philosophy why bother to inquire into others. The answer of course is that we suspect something is lacking in ours that we may find in the study of someone else's. It is the level of dissatisfaction with our own that triggers that search. Were we to be fairly content with our personal philosophy that we have evolved based on our life experiences, we would view the philosophy of others as merely of academic interest appropriate for a university faculty. It follows that, if everyone were fairly satisfied with his or her own views of life, whether or not able to fully implement them, philosophy as an academic study might become of historical interest only.

cosmopolitan (Judeo-Christian) and active today via the human conscience. But Isagorial Theory does more than identify the evils of transgression on others. It identifies the primary problem, which is not the individual. It is, instead, authoritarian governance and the transgressions it makes on the individual. It shows that when that authoritarianism is blocked freedom will lead to success of the entrepreneurial group and the community as a whole will prosper. Replace authoritarian governance and there will be little need for philosophy-derived correctives.

It is relevant to note that John Lewis, the prominent historian and Objectivist scholar, once pointed out in a lecture on Objectivism that its logical composition, like any well-developed philosophy, is complete and perfect, and that a single discrepancy in principle can bring down the entire structure.[15] But the underlying mechanism of Isagorial Theory is malleable and adjustable by degrees. A little bit of freedom is better than none and a lot of freedom is better that a little bit. There is no "all or none" involved. All that needs be said is that the greater the civil liberty, the better the outcome, at least for human progress as judged by medical practice. And if human progress continues to improve mankind's condition there will be less competition for life's graces, a more secure and content population will be more tolerant and will better manage the planet, and fewer philosophies will be needed to provide excuses for contentious ideas.

Furthermore, implementation of Isagorial Theory would provide opportunity for any person in a society to work in his or her self-interest. In contrast, within a society the reach of Objectivism as a philosophy is restricted to the interested individual, and in most societies they will be uncommon. Isagorial Theory is universal in its relevance and accessibility.

Isagorial Theory of Human Progress is a function of a group, not an individual. It is the combination of varying talents that is the engine for its success in furthering human progress by harnessing the ideas of several persons who are working in concert for self-betterment. Objectivism on the other hand, as a personal philosophy, is not a mechanism for human progress. It is conducive to progress, and the inventions and constructions of its heroes in Rand's novels exemplify the useful offspring of their efforts. Nevertheless, simple mathematics will show that the varied ideas of the small group when compared to the single idea of a lone individual, is going to be more efficient in identifying, implementing and amplifying those ideas.

Lastly, Isagorial Theory and its association with Judeo-Christianity spans generations and even civilizations, whereas Objectivism has visited but two generations and will only make its presence felt in sympathetic societies. In other words, Isagorial Theory is relevant in any age, whereas Objectivism is relevant only now. It requires a modern society with significant individual freedom that allows Objectivism to take advantage of what freedom has already produced. It has, nevertheless, an important role to be played in preventing the deterioration of modern society. Although it may argue that it has no intentions regarding the course of society, it should, because unless it does get involved it may end up in no better position than pacifist Quakers, who, when the State is in complete control of society, will be among the first to be regulated into anonymity.

---

[15] This was also stated in a 1985 lecture by Dr. Peikoff: "If anything is wrong anywhere, anybody who is interested in the truth should correct it. Does that mean that I concede that maybe there is an essential principle of Objectivism that is wrong? No, because by my understanding for the reason I just told you, it's one totality. So if any one principle is wrong, the whole thing is collapsed."

Conclusion

Objectivism and Isagorial Theory of Human Progress are, in most areas, consistent with natural law, its Judeo-Christian expression, and each other, the former operating through the individual and the latter through the group. Despite resistance to acknowledging the relevance of Judeo-Christianity, Objectivism performs in accordance with natural law and for this reason is a virtuous philosophy (see Excursus 4) despite lack of any religious motive. Furthermore, Objectivism does not restrict humaneness in any way. Both Objectivism and Isagorial Theory favor self-betterment and freedom; the former demands it as a personal philosophy, and the latter declares it necessary for human progress. Moreover, the beneficent consequences of their self-interest can extend to include the common good even though unintended, and this also is a virtuous act even in the absence of motive. Although it is only Isagorial Theory that has been proven (in *The Natural State of Medical Practice*) to facilitate the initiation and maturation of human progress, the personal philosophy of Objectivism is capable of promoting and contributing to it. There would seem to be a natural association between the two if someone would but try. But the practical distinction between the two remains: Objectivism is an attractive and valuable personal philosophy, whereas Isagorial Theory has (1) identified the nemesis that has made Objectivism broadly attractive and (2) exposes a cosmopolitan strategy to defeat it.

As a final comment, aspects of this excursus remind me of my childhood dentist in Ada, Ohio, who, while explaining the importance of preventive dentistry to his ten-year-old patient, acknowledged that his ultimate professional goal was to put himself out of business. Perhaps it is asking too much of Objectivists to join forces with Judeo-Christianity and the Isagorial Theory of Human Progress in their battle.

EXCURSUS 11

This is an explanatory monograph on the purpose and significance of the message presented on the **contratyrannos.com** website of the Isagorial Theory of Human Progress. That theory, derived from *The Natural State of Medical Practice*, is not about herbal therapies, alternative medicine, or the beauties of primitivism. It does not promote any inherent ethnic or geographic superiority in advancing human progress. Nor, in its references to the "common man and woman," is it an attempt to instigate a rebellion among the disadvantaged. It is, instead, a warning to everyone of danger to human progress that lies ahead, a warning exposed by this social history of medical practice as interpreted by a physician.

PRESSING IMPLICATIONS OF THE NATURAL STATE OF MEDICAL PRACTICE[1]

The problem and its history

We are living in a unique time when the global population is broadly benefiting from the freedoms of the common man and woman in the West, freedoms traceable to the Reformation. For the first time in human history the greater part of a civilization has escaped its authoritarian cage and enjoyed an extended period of natural rights protection. But given the tragic history of mankind over thousands of years as revealed in *The Natural State of Medical Practice*, it is critical to prevent a repetition of the carnage.

That carnage has been stark indeed. In the Epilogue to volume 3 of *The Natural State of Medical Practice* an estimate of the number of humans that have existed since the first man and woman, dated from 50,000 BC to modern times, is about one hundred billion. Some may view my inclusion of this coarse estimate of the entirety of humankind as a rhetorical prank, but that is not the case. It is, instead, to further impress on readers the unimaginable but true level of tragedy for a mankind without effective medical care, a world incomprehensible to the younger Western generation of today. That is, one hundred billion individuals like you. We may like to believe that, except for specific wars, pogroms, and natural disasters we read about in history books, people departed this life in bed for the most part with loved ones nearby and a kind and caring shaman or the equivalent in attendance, whether in caves, tepees, cabins or Dickensian tenements. This was surely not the case. Misery abounded especially for the unprivileged, or common citizenry, mortality was mostly unexpected because it occurred in a young population,[2]

---

[1] Volume, chapter and page number of otherwise unreferenced statements in this monograph refer to the version of the three volumes as published by Liberty Hill Press in 2019:

　Vol. 1 – *The Natural State of Medical Practice: An Isagorial Theory of Human Progress*
　Vol. 2 – *The Natural State of Medical Practice: Hippocratic Evidence*
　Vol. 3 - *The Natural State of Medical Practice: Escape from Egalitarianism*

The epidemiological support for many claims in this excursus is found in volumes 1 and 3.

[2] Life expectancy for the mass of mankind remained little more than thirty years until the last two hundred years. Supporting data are present in *The Natural State of Medical Practice*, volume 1, and in Excursus 3.

for relief from pain there was little or nothing, and for most of those hundred billion it was fear of death, not love of life, that prompted human survival, that plus sexuality. For 49,700 of the 50,000 years of human history and prehistory there can be found no uplifting vision of humanity with its ups and downs on some inevitable path of improvement in medical care. The cartoonish implication that, from the four-legged *Proconsul africanus* or ape-like creature to placing a man on the moon, humanity has gradually but inevitably and permanently arrived, courtesy of a superior brain, at its well-deserved zenith, that "the universe is unfolding as it should," is a bad joke. Admittedly a few placid lacunae blessed the ruling classes. But for the rest of us, it has been an unchanging spectacle of anguish, whether it be the pain and agony as seen in wide-eyed innocent babies, in the questioning anxiety of the febrile dyspneic child, in the frightened adolescent (whether from mortally obstructed labor of a primigravida or the unanticipated helplessness of lethal illness), in a delirious young adult with a mortal injury or battle wound, or in the saddened older adult, most under forty years of age, recognizing the inevitable.

The cause of the problem

In *The Natural State of Medical Practice* two sources are identified as causes for this depressing history of mankind: in prehistory it was social egalitarianism of the tribe and in history it has been the politics of power. Both are the public face of authoritarian governance.

An authoritarian society seems invincible for two reasons: it is efficient and it is ruthless. It is also difficult to root out because it insinuates itself into all aspects of life, and, as identified by Alexis de Tocqueville, making it difficult to leave for reasons of security, safety and suspicion.[3] This process is facilitated by controlling dissent and propagandizing. With the birth of the United States of America, however, those mechanisms have shown themselves to be vulnerable, for a free society was now proven capable on its own of fashioning a mechanism for freedom and security of the individual despite restraining political power, and history has shown the American experiment to result in prosperity and progress for all its citizens.

At its core the issue is power, or, to be more specific, centralization of power in government. That centralization may be acquired by force or guile, or it may be gifted to a central government by members of society in return for favors. Just as the 16th C Vatican enriched and empowered itself by sanctioning preprinted indulgences for the influential, centralized secular governance, whether despotic or democratic, will do the same and over time will concentrate authority in fewer and fewer hands and further restrict natural rights. The process inevitably involves purposeful imposition of targeted areas of ignorance (censorship) for the general population, and government's bad decisions and low opinion of the value of the now ignorant "common" people and their expendability in promoting the State can easily lead to conflict. Almost ninety percent of the Russian army in World War I in 1917 were peasants (total Russian military deaths: 1.8 million), and six hundred thousand young Chinese men were killed or wounded in the Korean War (1950-1953) because Mao Zedong desired to increase the prestige of China in the communist world.

---

[3] See: de Tocqueville, A., *Democracy in America*, New York, 1946, vol. 2, pp. 335, 336, for this predicted trend in America.

The solution to the problem

And this brings us to the purpose of this excursus, maintaining that freedom. Alarmingly, a malignant process of gifting the personal freedom of the unprivileged men and women of society to centralized authoritarian governance is rapidly occurring in modern society. The appeal of this website is, therefore, to the unprivileged citizenry, to resist that process. But first, who are the common man and woman?

It is to be made clear from the beginning that the **contratyrannos.com** website does not recognize any man and woman as "common." The variation in abilities distributed throughout humankind exists for a reason, and that reason is to improve our condition in life. I am aware of teleological issues regarding causation, but the fact remains, human variation is real, universal, and serves a purpose. We are not meant to be like a colony of ants. It is logical, therefore, that to exclude a percent of members of a society from their attempting self-betterment is an existential threat not only for that segment of society but for the entirety of society as well.

For it is from the general pool of the common citizenry, not its elected or self-appointed leaders, that good things flow. And we praise peculiar genius and its beneficences to Western society, but we should be aware that genius abounds in every age and every society and in some guise and in some degree is present in every person. And that concept of "every person" is unqualified, not imagined or rhetorical. Throughout the existence of humankind, the serfs, the enslaved, the prematurely dying, the enforced infirmities, the ninety percent of the European population purposefully ensnared in medieval bondage, the eighty percent of the Russian 19th C population that were peasants, and the eighty million poor peasants of the 15th C Ming Dynasty, included in their lot not only Newtons, Shakespeares, Bachs, Michelangelos and Einsteins, but also the myriad different expressions of genius that, depending on personal motives, priorities, chance or opportunity, might have appeared in the work of individuals in those populations but were purposefully prevented from emerging.

For, as shown in these volumes, the modern medical and thereby many related scientific advances that have so improved the life of modern society are the product of no elite class nor done under the direction of an elite class, instead being the spontaneous consequences of a (relatively) free society that has permitted the inherent and broad genius within society to reveal itself and to finally do, or at least begin to do, what was intended be done. Mankind's progress can be attributed *entirely* to absence of governance, period. And it is because American governance, building on post-Reformation political changes in the West and especially in the Netherlands and England, was so wonderfully designed to protect the natural rights and forbidden to intrude into the lives of its citizens that prompted America's intellectual dominance in the world within little more than a century of its founding.

The "common" citizenry herein are not those who would man the barricades to demand their share of the bounties of modern society. Instead, in the centuries following the Reformation they demanded their freedoms and their opportunity to exploit their uncommonness for their own benefit. And once released from feudal bondage and pan-European theocratic kinship, they proved their greater worth in the West as those bounties naturally transferred to the greater society. There was no stimulus for such a remarkable transition; none was needed. It is natural and inherent to attempt to overcome an adversity. And their benefit to society was not directed by any authority for the direction was not known, and, as with Hippocratic medicine of ancient Greece, that authority often was fortuitously occupied elsewhere. Given the ability to proceed, a free people will not make demands on others when they are free to make do on their own. No credit can be given to preexisting governance, for no governance will diminish its control and power if left to its own devices. *In a word, no governance can claim to have contributed to human progress.*

But authoritarianism in any form requires constant attention to persist. It is unnatural, and in a sense its leaders and admirers know it. To continue to exist it must continuously accumulate and maintain power at any cost, and its primary tool is manipulation of the general population. If this ceases, the whole thing falls apart.

And that is curious. A society released from authoritarian bondage may fragment, but it does not atomize. The fragments quickly find a way to come together and begin to prosper, as seen in the settlement hierarchies of ancient primary city-states as described in *The Natural State of Medical Practice* and in post-World War democracies. And those today who escape from totalitarian States promptly relish their freedoms in Western democracies. People inculcated in their formative years with State propaganda inevitably reside comfortably in the West without governance shaping all their decisions. And so it is that, barring replacement of one kind of authoritarianism with another, a land that recognizes natural rights will win. That is, unless it reneges on the guarantee of those rights. And it is this that must be perpetually protected, for never has there been a government unwilling to so renege.

A freedom-loving citizenry promotes progress and improvement in the human condition, and when left alone it is like a self-righting ship: remove authoritarian restrictions and the citizens will set things aright. If the central power structure of the Chinese Communist Party were to disappear and be prevented from reorganizing in the various provinces, a peaceful revolution would be reflected in improvements in the human condition throughout the region, one based on the inherent genius of its citizens rather than on recent governmental slight-of-hand that has merely allowed its people to prosper by imitating the fruits of genius of free citizens in the West.

Concluding and qualifying comments:

(1) The world and our immediate political environment are what they are, and to completely exchange the immediate with the desired is fanciful. It will take time and tenacity to peel back the levels of dependency that have accumulated on the citizenry over the past century. It is also naïve to think that the desired goal will ever be reached, for arguments will be as endless as are human opinions on everything. For this reason the seemingly black and white problems relevant to progress or serfdom for humanity presented in **contratyrannos.com** should be recognized for what they are: simplified illustrations and conclusions derived from observations of complicated societies. There is, however, one strong argument in its favor: *The Natural State of Medical Practice* offers a proof of the existence and a qualitative estimate of the danger of authoritarian governance by recounting the unimaginable tragedy in human history that has resulted from its willful efforts at control.

(2) It is central to the idea of the Isagorial Theory of Human Progress that the causes of all the major problems in society are found in governance alone, not the people. If governance over time is matched to conform with human civil liberty and natural rights,

there would be simultaneous cessation of much contentious discussion and threats. And this is because threats emanating from governance itself would cease. At the same time the broadly disseminated genius of *Homo sapiens* working in self-interest would generally assert itself to the unintended benefit of everyone. There is a natural morality (natural law) inherent in every person.

(3) It is not a corollary of this work that there should be freedom from man-made laws that are necessary for an ordered society. And there must be laws to protect natural rights from infringements, for the distinction between right and wrong is often uncertain and issues of crime and punishment require judgment within a humane society. Then there are issues that extend beyond those affecting one or a few members of society, instead being a threat to all, that, whether of a military or other existential nature, can require broad debate or speedy action.

(4) The present works have been derived from study of the history of medical practice, and it is merely an assumption that they are relevant to other areas of great societal interest, such as physics, economics and biology. On the other hand, the rise to prominence of the West concurrently with remarkable progress of medical care suggests a general usefulness of the Isagorial Theory of Human Progress (and see Excursus 18). But there is no theory that would not benefit from more study.

(5) The conclusions of this work, originally targeting medical practice but suggested as being of general relevance, will not be applicable within authoritarian governance. The Isagorial Theory of Human Progress itself will be irrelevant when elements of democracy do not exist. And this is the great question in view of the trend to globalization in a world increasingly controlled by autocratic and authoritarian governments. A centralized global authority governing economic and commercial interests will doom the theory, along with freedom itself.

6) It is pointed out in *The Natural State of Medical Practice* that the Isagorial Theory of Human Progress is not a philosophy (and see Excursus 10). It is, instead, an interpretation of facts of history that illuminates the path to human progress. As such, its effectiveness in that illumination is not like an all-or-none contract, and, unlike a philosophy, its perceived effectiveness does not require perfection in implementation. In effect, a little bit is better than none and a lot is better than some. No revolutionary change is necessary to implement it, with the exception that its task is to minimize authoritarian controls.

(7) One might ask why we in the free world are not flooded with genius if everyone has the potential for genius (defined as "great natural ability;" Merriam-Webster). Reasons include personal priorities such as family duties, preference for time with family, extensive responsibilities, passion for one's regular job or pastime, volunteering time and effort, inhospitable residential environments, expressions of genius known only to oneself or to a limited circle of acquaintances, no opportunity to express the particular form of genius that one has, and so on. For all of these preoccupations that can eclipse overt expression of genius there is an element of personal choice. The issue is, instead, those malignant external agencies that actively prevent expression of natural genius on a large scale where it might otherwise appear, albeit unpredictably.

(8) And, finally, it must be clearly understood that the enemy is authoritarianism and its immoral attack on natural rights. Authoritarianism is not an abstract political or philosophical construct, one among many, such as Marxism, Nietzscheanism, Existentialism and Hegelianism, "isms" that academics interpret in various ways. It is also to be made clear that the history of mankind reveals that authoritarianism has never lost a battle. Only in the modern West has it been held in abeyance, and that resistance is

clearly weakening as the inherent efficiency of the enforced unity of authoritarianism threatens the unenforceable diversity of a free citizenry. Do not forget that in the game on display the authoritarian disguises his true nature. The trap is ready to be sprung.

EXCURSUS 12

Following a formal validation of Isagorial Theory, the unintended consequences of authoritarian interference in society's natural rights are shown to reside in big government, thus giving us the warning:

> From him who sees no wood for trees,
> And yet is busie as the bees
> From him that's settled on his lees
> And speaketh not without his fees,
> Libera nos."[1]

VALIDATION OF THE ISAGORIAL THEORY OF HUMAN PROGRESS

Sumer	Egypt	India	China	Greece
Medical Treatise	*Papyrus Ebers*	*Charaka Samhita*	*Su Wen*	*Hippocratic Corpus*
2900 BC	3100 BC	2000 BC	2000 BC	600 BC
Early urbanization	Early urbanization	Urban	Early urbanization	Early urbanization
2350 BC	2600 BC	500 BC	300 BC	300 BC
Akkadian assimilation	Pharaonic assimilation	Hindu assimilation	Bureaucratic assimilation	Destabilization
Incorporation	Incorporation	Incorporation	Incorporation	
Disappearance	Disappearance	Ayurvedic Medicine	Traditional Chinese Medicine	Disappearance

This Table lists, in sequence, the regions, the critical medical texts, approximate or proposed date of origin of their rational clinical content, the social environments at that time, approximate dates of authoritarian intercession, the causes of that cessation, its mechanism, and ultimate status. Its purpose is to summarize the course of medical progress in human history that supports a proof for the Isagorial Theory of Human Progress.

Introduction

No, despite the crafty proverb of Mr. Heywood in 1546 I do not intend to diminish the significance of the work of the vast army of historians who over the centuries have conscientiously attempted to describe and interpret the history of mankind. Indeed, the theory I will now summarize is based on their careful labors. But it is my opinion that from the vast treasure they have recovered it is now possible to see the "forest" if we but

---

[1] A Letany for St. Omers, 1682, from: *Proverbs of John Heywood. Being the "Proverbes" of that author printed in 1546*, J. Sharman, ed., London, 1874.

step back and view the panorama in which the many battles of humankind have been fought. And it is my hope, therefore, that *The Natural State of Medical Practice* will be interpreted not as a historical recounting of a cornucopia of individual successes of our favorite predecessors but as a revelation and warning of panoramic failure.

The conclusions of *The Natural State of Medical Practice* rely on the correct interpretation of historical data surrounding the appearance and then disappearance of arguably nascent scientific medical practices in the ancient civilizations of Mesopotamia, Egypt, India, China, and Greece. These civilizations were initially studied because each began as a primary civilization and we possess ancient medical documents from each that have been acclaimed by scholars as consistent with those practices.[2] Conclusions from their study are the basis for the *Isagorial Theory of Human Progress* that is derived from it.[3] The documents are:

> Mesopotamia – *Treatise of Medical Diagnosis and Prognosis*
> Egypt – *Papyrus Ebers*
> India – *Charaka Samhita*
> China – *Huang Ti Nei Ching Su Wen*
> Ancient Greece – *Hippocratic Corpus*

Each is considered the foundational medical document for its respective civilization. Notably, of all the documents it is only the Egyptian *Papyrus Ebers* that in its original form may have included supernatural content, although even this is uncertain.

Thus, the scope of investigation of *The Natural State of Medical Practice* that led to the Isagorial Theory of Human Progress comprises medical practices from around the world. Its definition is:

> A theory ascribing all apolitical advances for the betterment of mankind to autonomous associations pursuing self-betterment in which each member has equal opportunity to speak freely and share ideas about the group's common interest without fear of retribution. Axiomatically it excludes "betterments" that have been stolen, copied, derived by exploitation, or used for subjugation of others.

Inevitably, investigative results attempt to be comprehensive, and profound generalizations will be based on an ocean of specific events and details. As in all objective studies that rely on data there will be outliers that do not fit into an all-inclusive generalization. Exceptions are found in everything, and it is with statistics that we attempt to focus on those things deemed most important. The Isagorial Theory of Human Progress entails both issues. On the one hand it is based on broad generalizations; on the other there is a rudimentary attempt at statistical analysis (see Appendix A, volume 1, of *The Natural State of Medical Practice*) in the hope that some of the outlying material can be reasonably excluded. It is my hope, therefore, that its conclusions will prompt others to apply to other essential subjects a similar analysis to test the validity of the Isagorial Theory of Human Progress.

---

[2] Definition of a "primary civilization:" A civilization that has not been "shaped by substantial dependence upon or control by other, more complex societies." (Trigger, B. G., *Understanding Early Civilizations,* Cambridge (UK), 2003, p. 19.)

[3] Also see: Majno, G., *The Healing Hand,* 1991, 1st paperback edition. This is an excellent clinical interpretation of medical practices in ancient civilizations and includes all five of the civilizations discussed in this excursus.

But first, a "theory" is, at its core and according to Merriam-Webster, a "supposition." That supposition is "based on general principles" independent of what is being supposed. The Cambridge Dictionary agrees: "a statement … based or suggested to explain a fact or event … or an opinion or explanation." The Stanford Encyclopedia of Philosophy definition of theory(s) is, in contrast, exceedingly complex. It is best, therefore, to focus on a practical definition of "theory" for a specific issue, and a convenient one is found in *Science News for Students* and can be summarized as *an explanation of how something happens based on experiments, observations and facts that have been confirmed.*

Using the latter definition, the Isagorial Theory of Human Progress (herein the "Theory"), to be considered a valid theory that can be taken as a serious attempt to explain the course and causes of success and failure of human progress, should depend on confirmed facts and observations. How closely does the Theory adhere to this requirement?

1. Factual basis of the Theory - The Theory is derived from the facts of history as provided in scientific journals and books by hundreds of scholars. I am not a historian and am not competent to judge the factuality of historical events uncovered by specialists who often have disparate views of the same event. I have tried to consider and to include competing views in developing the Theory. Ancient history, however, is fraught with inconsistent judgments regarding facts, and even basic factual information concerning dates, names, and locations is often unavailable and therefore is often an estimate or guess, however insightful.

2. Observational basis of the Theory – This means the actual observation of something by someone, which in the realm of history usually is a personal observation by a participant or bystander or a relevant contemporary description of an event that is generally held by those affected by the event. It often is unavoidably subjective, and a corollary is the myth or legend arising from the event that has become a virtual fact in the minds of contemporaries and descendants but which has little basis in fact. In some situations, however, there may indeed have been a factual basis underlying the origin of the myth or legend. This is discussed in volume 3 of *The Natural State of Medical Practice,* p. 31.[4]

Given the scientific limitations of historical theories as outlined above, the historical observations and facts upon which the Isagorial Theory of Human Progress is based can now be reviewed. Three arguments representing the basis for its conclusions are presented: **(1) The credibility of basic documents** upon which the arguments rest should be considered consistent with progress in the field of medicine according to modern medical judgment rather than contemporary or popular opinion; **(2) There should be evidence for early urbanization** as the social environment that permitted the initiation of medical progress, a phase sometimes referred to as a "settlement hierarchy;"[5] **(3) Evidence of authoritarian manipulation** should explain the loss or termination of that

---

[4] Also see: Honko, L., *The Problem of Defining Myth*, in *Sacred Narrative*, Alan Dundes, ed., Berkeley, 1984, pp.41-52, especially p. 45.

[5] Definition of a settlement hierarchy: "A natural progression of intergroup adjustments that spontaneously occurs as an urbanizing society, having no prior experience with a political hierarchy, becomes more complex and acquires facilities, goods and services to accommodate an enlarging population." A "primary city-state" is an early city-state that is not a colony and is unaffiliated with a larger civilization.

medical progress. These three arguments are now reviewed as they apply to each of the five civilizations.

Elaboration on arguments supporting the Theory

First, there is an axiomatic base upon which the Theory rests. The following points are made and explained in *The Natural State of Medical Practice*:

1. The initial steps leading to medical discovery are cheap, easy, quick, simple, and at hand. No technology is required. In medicine we call this the history and physical examination of the patient.
2. The steps leading to scientific medical discovery require a group of practitioners and a large population under observation for, to be scientific, a discovery needs confirmation. Each person responds uniquely to an illness or injury, and, except for epidemics, illness and injury tend to be sporadic and at best only modestly predictable. A sporadic medical event, therefore, is better confirmed within the combined experience of a group of practitioners acting within a large population. An observation within one's family circle or tribe may be correct, but to be scientific it needs confirmation. A minimum requirement based on a limited statistical analysis is proposed in *The Natural State of Medical Practice*, volume 3, Appendix A, for initiation of a sustainable medical profession capable of maintaining medical progress over time: a collegial association of at least three or four practitioners in a prosperous and politically stable region and an accessible population in the range of ten thousand.

Thus, even without knowledge of their origin, the medical documents upon which the validity of the Theory is based can, with reasonable confidence, be declared the work of at least several practitioners working collegially in the midst of a large population rather than a single practitioner moving from village to village. This should be reflected in the social environment of the time.

Mesopotamia:

Credible document: The medical document most studied by medical and linguistic scholars has been the Sumerian *Treatise of Medical Diagnosis and Prognosis*. The prescient nature of its knowledge is described in articles written by medical subspecialists and is especially well outlined in the excellent book by Drs. Scurlock and Andersen, the latter a specialist in infectious diseases, and works of other scholars.[6] In addition to these references, I comment in *The Natural State of Medical Practice*, volume 3, pp. 53-54, that a procedure described to drain fluid from the chest had to be based on the experience of many practitioners over time, thus adding to the argument for a Sumerian collegial medical affiliation of some sort.

---

[6] See: Scurlock, J., and Andersen, B. R., *Diagnoses in Assyrian and Babylonian Medicine*, Chicago, 2005; Paullisian, R.; *Medicine in Ancient Assyria and Babylonia*, in *J. Assyrian Academic Studies*, 5:3-51, 1991.

Evidence for early urbanization: The evidence from medical sources, however minimal, is sufficient to confidently claim a significant formal medical presence existed during the Early Dynastic period of Sumer (2900-2350 BC) or earlier, perhaps in the Jemdet Nasr period (3100-2900 BC) of the prosperous city-state of Uruk, population 50,000, prior to domination and unification of the regional Sumerian city-states by the Akkadian monarch, Sargon (24th C BC).[7] There of course had been no prior experience with a medical profession. If 2900 BC is chosen as the approximate dating of this evidence it would be late in the "settlement hierarchy" phase of urbanization of Uruk.[8]

Evidence for authoritarian manipulation: Although Sumerian medicine was admired and some of the texts of scholarly works would be transmitted in Sumerian cuneiform for two thousand years, the degradation of the clinical practitioner paralleled the centralization of political power in Mesopotamia during subsequent troubled times. The degradation of the *azu* (physician) commenced with the appearance of the exorcist-priest, *asipu*, of the early Akkadian conquerors (*ca.* 2300 BC). Payment for the *azu* was then regulated by the Code of Ur-Nammu (2050 BC), and penalties for errors of the *azu* were imposed by the Code of Hammurabi (1750 BC). The *azu* is not even mentioned for centuries in the monarchical regimes following the Old Babylonian period. In contrast, the *asipu* became increasingly prominent over these centuries, using the early clinical wisdom of the *azu* in the *Treatise of Medical Diagnosis and Prognosis* while contributing none of his own. Omens, while common in Akkadian, are absent in writings from earlier Sumer even though gods and goddesses were in abundance.[9] It is notable that the *azu* was again recognized in the militant Neo-Assyrian empire (911-609 BC), but only as a medical companion to retrieve the wounded during military actions. The exorcist *asipu*, in contrast, remained identifiable throughout all periods, even to the 4th C BC, and magic featured prominently in the subsequent medicine of Zoroastrianism of the Persian Empire (550-330 BC).

Egypt:

Credible document: There are a mere twelve medical papyri that grace the medicine of the 2600-year-old ancient Egyptian civilization, most of which deal heavily with magic and with repetitions of clinical sections from the singular *Papyrus Ebers*, which therefore

---

[7] The Sumerian medical practitioner (the *azu*) is mentioned as early as 2900 BC, and the Electronic Text Corpus of Sumerian Literature (ETCSL) at the University of Oxford provides a text concerning a goddess, Ninisina A, who is described as a healer, a helper for childbirth, and possessor of a scalpel (t.4.22.1). This goddess, holding a scalpel, is first attested in Early Dynasty IIIa (2600-2450), although her earlier manifestation is thought to be Ninsun (or Ninisina) the mother of Gilgamesh, now considered an early king of the Early Dynastic city-state of Uruk (?Isin, *ca.* 2800 BC). It is to be admitted, however, that the two earliest extant rational Sumerian cuneiform tablets date only from *ca.* 2500 BC in the western Sumerian city of Ebla, although they presumably reflect pre-existing earlier rational medicine in a central Sumerian city-state such as Uruk. Furthermore, it probably took two or three centuries for a professional medical component to evolve to the point that it could be so highly regarded as to be assigned to a goddess.

[8] It has been stated that the settlement hierarchy phase and the political centralization phase of urbanization can co-exist for extended periods, and evidence suggests no rigid political hierarchy existed at the time of Gilgamesh.

[9] Michalowski, P., *How to Read the Liver – in Sumerian*, in *If a Man Builds a Joyful House*, A. K. Guinan, *et al.*, eds., Leiden 2006, pp. 247-258,

must be considered the pinnacle of ancient Egyptian medical scholarship. Much scholarship has centered on ancient Egyptian medicine as a forerunner of Western modern medicine, and excellent translations and commentary have revealed the valuable clinical detail of *Papyrus Ebers* and its near contemporary, the Edwin Smith papyrus.[10] Both are acclaimed as works of great medical insight.[11]

Evidence of early urbanization: An inscription in the 16th C BC copy of *Papyrus Ebers* states that it (meaning the original version) was shown to the 1st Dynasty pharaoh, Den, whose rule is presently dated 3000 to 2960 BC (found in paragraph 856a of the papyrus). Scholars have cautioned that the dating of *Papyrus Ebers* with the pharaoh Den should not be assumed to be correct.[12] On the other hand, the *Berlin Medical Papyrus* of the 18th Dynasty contains much that is in *Papyrus Ebers* and a similar mention of Pharaoh Den.[13] The *Papyrus of Ani* of the 19th Dynasty contains elements that have been described as "primeval," validating the possibility of even predynastic material finding its way into later papyri. The Wellcome Institute cites a page of the *Papyrus Ebers* that contains a recipe from the 1st dynasty. The 3rd C BC Egyptian historian, Manetho, cites the 1st dynasty pharaoh, Athothis, as a "physician" and author of an anatomical text. The social environment of Hierakonpolis as an autonomous Egyptian primary city-state in *ca.* 3100 BC has been reviewed, and its principal features are consistent with the settlement hierarchy phase of urbanization. It can be concluded that the clinical material in *Papyrus Ebers* comes from the Naqada III or 1st Dynastic period (together, 3200-2890 BC), probably the former.

Evidence for authoritarian manipulation: With centralization of power in the early centuries following the unification of Upper and Lower Egypt under the first pharaoh, the wisdom of the early practitioners became canonized and subsumed by priest-physicians of the palace beginning in the Old Kingdom period (2700-2200 BC). Medical progress not only ceased; it was increasingly magical and regressed. By the time of the Persian

---

[10] Allen, J. P., *The Art of Medicine in Ancient Egypt*, New York, 2005.

[11] For example: van Middendorp, J. J., Sanchez, G. M., and Burridge, A. L., The Edwin Smith Papyrus: A Clinical Reappraisal of the Oldest Known Document in Spinal Injuries, in *Eur. Spine J.*, 19:1815-1823, 2010; Strouhal, E., Vachala, B., and Vymazalova, H., *The Medicine of the Ancient Egyptians*, New York, 2014; Nunn, J. F. Ancient Egyptian Medicine, Norman (OK); Majno, G., *The Healing Hand*, Cambridge (MA), 1975.

[12] John Nunn: *Ancient Egyptian Medicine*, Norman (OK), 1996, p. 31

[13] That the original *Papyrus Ebers*, or its content, was seen by Den suggests the nascent Egyptian medical practitioner of his time had already acquired a good reputation above and beyond the reputation that circulates among one's kin and friends. Some estimate the date of the original *Papyrus Ebers* to be as early as 3400 BC, although the hieratic script of the papyrus was not developed until the Naqada III period (3200-3000 BC). As with the early Sumerian dating of its collection of clinical material, it is reasonable to estimate the Egyptian clinical observations were made during the two centuries preceding pharaoh Den, *i.e., ca.* 3200-3000 BC. In an autonomous primary city-state of the time (Hierakonpolis, settled in late 5th millennium BC) there was an increasing population and prosperity guided by a commercial heterarchy even though there were local leaders that were evolving an elite class. Kinship affiliations have been judged to be not prominent, and specialization in services and crafts proliferated. Prosperity and progress in medicine, as found in *Papyrus Ebers*, would continue into the Early Dynastic period, along with freedom of artistic expression among the non-elite population.

conquest (525 BC) nothing of significance remained. [14] Diodorus Siculus (1st C BC) then cited severe penalties should a "physician" deviate from the ancient Egyptian writings.

India:

Credible document: Essentials of the earliest medical practice in India are considered to reside in the Vedas, specifically the Rig Veda and the Atharva Veda. Their mature secular form is considered to be modern Ayurveda, with the medical classic, the *Charaka Samhita*, acclaimed as its initial masterwork. Underlying the many statements in that document that to the modern mind seem absurd, there is much clinical description documenting the prescience of many Indian practitioners in ages past. [15]

Evidence for relevance of early urbanization: Tradition has tied the wisdom of the *Charaka Samhita* (the "collection of Charaka") to the Vedic Age, 1500 to 500 BC by current scholarly estimations but probably prior to 2000 BC by some authorities, although the *Charaka Samhita* itself was probably physically compiled *ca.* 1st C BC. Its legendary (mythical?) author was Agnivesha in the 8th C BC. Charaka himself has yet to be specifically identified, but Dr. Chattopadhyaya has proposed the word "caraka," meaning "wanderer," to be closer to the truth. [16] This would equate the early Indian practitioners with the itinerant physicians of ancient Greece and China. But the basis for the rational medical knowledge of the *Charaka Samhita* is considered to be the Rig Veda, the oldest and most revered of the several Vedas and dated to the early years of the Vedic Age. The confidence with which its pronouncements about contemporary medical practitioners are made indicate a medical profession not only existed when Rig Veda was composed but had existed, and over a wide area, for some time, perhaps several centuries. Importantly, its medical statements contain no numinous component, whereas the much later *Charaka Samhita* has much mystical and religious content as well as additional advice from its subsequent non-physician editors. There is also no question but that the clinical content of the *Charaka Samhita* reflected the medical environment of a large population. The idea that it was cumulative experience arising from irregularly visiting hamlets and villages over a broad area by isolated, illiterate and competitive "wandering" practitioners is untenable. Sizeable Indian cities in ancient times belonged either to the Indus River Valley civilization (2600 to 1900 BC) or to the "second urbanization period" (500 to 200 BC). Only local populations surrounding separate and discrete monarchical centers of the subcontinent existed during the intervening centuries. [17] It is proposed, therefore, that the collection of clinical information was already available late in the 1st millennium BC when

---

[14] "There is no evidence of major changes in the format or content of classical Egyptian medicine between the Old Kingdom and the end of the Twenty-sixth Dynasty, covering the years 2600 to 525 BC... ." J. F. Nunn, in *Ancient Egyptian Medicine*, Norman (OK), 1996, p. 206.

[15] As Dr. Debriprasad Chattopadhyaya states, "... their great significance and reputation despite the heap of intellectual debris eventually piled upon them." *Science and Society in Ancient India*, Amsterdam, 1977.

[16] See the magisterial work of G. J. Muelenbeld, *A History of Indian Medical Literature*, volume Ia, Part 1, for an exhaustive account of the dates and identities of those who might have been affiliated with the original *Charaka Samhita*. But I rely much on Dr. Chattopadhyaya's insightful book in the previous footnote.

[17] In his list of largest cities, Tertius Chandler lists no subcontinent large cities between 1900 and 500 BC: *Four Thousand Years of Urban Growth:* An Historical Census, Wales, 1987.

Hinduism formally emerged. The only possible site for its origin is the extraordinary Indus River Valley civilization with its many large cities. One of its larger, autonomous and prosperous city-states was Mohenjo Daro, located in present-day southern Pakistan. Its archeological structure was egalitarian and there is no evidence of centralized political power.

Evidence for authoritarian manipulation: Beginning about 2000 BC, and presumably because of climate change rather than conquest, Indus River Valley cities declined, their population moving primarily toward the east. Many centuries later it was the Brahmin caste of Hinduism that, being the most scholarly of the Varna system, involved itself in the work of the ancient Indian medical practitioners. From perhaps the 5th C BC to the 5th C AD Brahmins were involved in medical practice and the education of those who would be practitioners. Their scholars, presumably including Charaka and Drdhabala, the 5th C AD editor, compiled and edited, respectively, the *Charaka Samhita* and added numinous content from Hinduism so that the collected work came to be seen as a Vedic classic integral to Hindu tradition. But later in the 1st millennium AD the association of Brahmins with medical practitioners came to an end as medicine was viewed as a low caste purview.[18] As part of the canon of Hinduism, there has been no clinical progress in Ayurveda beyond the mere recovery of some of its ancient edited content as found in the *Charaka Samhita,* although periodically new botanical observations occurred.

China:

Credible document: The *Huang Ti Nei Ching Su Wen*, translated by Dr. Veith as *The Yellow Emperor's Classic of Internal Medicine*, has been uniformly considered the masterwork of Chinese medicine for centuries.[19] Its authority has extended to today's Traditional Chinese Medicine. First documented in an early bibliographic catalogue of the Han Dynasty (the Qilue, 2nd C BC), it received a major editing and amending by the non-physician, Wang Bing, in the 8th C AD. This has been the source of the modern version of the text. Its core tenets include the uniqueness of the individual patient and a non-mystical approach to causation and therapy. There are many reasonable and insightful clinical observations, and it is universally agreed that it is the work of many practitioners, although whether there was a collegial association is not mentioned.

Evidence for relevance of early urbanization: Traditional thinking has the *Huang Ti Nei Ching Su Wen* dated to the time of Huang Ti, the Yellow Emperor, the legendary (? mythical) unifier of early China *ca.* 2500 BC. Scholars do not accept this as factual, and most would put its compilation of medical wisdom about 300 BC, with the majority of its

---

[18] Hunter, W. W., *The Indian Empire: Its People, History and Products*, New Delhi, 2005, a reprint of the 1886 original, p. 109. This work was apparently translated and used in contemporary schools in India.

[19] See: Veith, I., *The Yellow Emperor's Classic of Internal Medicine*, Baltimore, 1949. Her work included only 32 of the 81 chapters of the *Huang Ti Nei Ching Su Wen.*

content being contemporary" but with the clinical core possibly much older.[20,21] The Han Dynasty (202 BC-220 AD) mention of the *Huang Ti Nei Ching Su Wen* in the Qilue bibliography of extant books indicates its knowledge was already ancient. There is no evidence of medical practitioners in the intervening Xia and Shang dynasties (2070-1050 BC) even though the Chinese writing was evolving and referred to oracles and shamans. The Zhou dynasty (1050-256 BC), in the Rites of Zhou (*ca.* 260 BC) mentions palace "physicians" with seemingly paramedical tasks but no knowledgeable treatise. It is proposed, therefore, that the social environment of the Shandong Longshan Culture of the legendary Yellow Emperor provided the clinical foundation of the *Huang Ti Nei Ching Su Wen*. Of the few population centers of the time, one of the largest was Liangchengzhen, notable for its lack of centralized commercial regulation and located near the coast. I propose it is from such an early population center as Liangchengzhen in the late Longshan period, *ca.* 2000 BC, prior to the invention of writing and at a time when urban specialists in goods and services first appeared, that medical practitioners first entered into collegial affiliations and acquired the medical knowledge that would later be the basis for the *Huang Ti Nei Ching Su Wen*.[22] It would be passed down orally in fragments for centuries before being an acknowledged comprehensive medical treatise during the Han dynasty.

Evidence for authoritarian manipulation: Whatever the resolution of the origin of rational medical wisdom found in the *Huang Ti Nei Ching Su Wen*, the wisdom itself, as codified and amended by Wang Bing, a nonphysician, in the 8th C AD, did not evolve. Once bureaucratically entrapped and canonized, the clinical knowledge of the *Huang Ti Nei Ching Su Wen* would never improve, as indicated by its veneration even today. Instead, the only aspect of ancient Chinese medicine that increased was its botanical menagerie of medicinal herbs and other substances. Dynastic emperors over subsequent centuries commissioned massive herbals from information gleaned throughout their empires, usually collected and compiled by non-physicians, but scientific merit was not sought, even into the 20th century, when it was reintroduced by the Chinese People's Republic as Traditional Chinese Medicine, a cheap but inferior alternative to Western medicine.

---

[20] Unschuld, P., *Medicine in China: A History of Ideas*, Berkeley, 2010, the 25th anniversary edition, p. 25.

[21] Ma, B., *A History of Medicine in Chinese Culture*, Singapore, 2020. It should be mentioned that there is a public site identified as the birthplace of Emperor Huang Ti, and elsewhere footprints attributed to him have been preserved.

[22] It has been noted by scholars that the *Rites of Zhou* from the late Warring States period (475-221 BC) contains elements of bureaucratic structure traceable to the Duke of Zhou (the "honorable and virtuous king" who reigned 1042-1035 BC) because the compilers of the *Rites of Zhou* included venerable bureaucratic structures of the Duke of Zhou so as to make their new bureaucratic system more acceptable to critics. Analogously, perhaps the Warring States historians who some propose to have compiled the *Huang Ti Nei Ching Su Wen* retained fragments of orally transmitted knowledge from the Longshan Culture in their compilation because any association with the Yellow Emperor (Huang Ti) would be considered venerable authentication of their work. As writing and collegial medical affiliations tend to occur contemporaneously, I predict that at some point in the archeology of Liangchengzhen or similar Longshan population center early Chinese characters referring to medical practitioners will be found. That a preceding form of writing existed in the region, see the evidence by Dr. Paolo Dematte in *The Origins of Chinese Writing: The Neolithic Evidence*, in *Cambridge Archaeological Journal*, 20:221-228, 2010.

Ancient Greece:

Credible document: Documented far beyond any other ancient system of medicine, the Hippocratic Corpus remains today a respected source of information on all aspects of clinical medicine, as well as the Hippocratic Oath. It still provides us with surprising insights.[23]

Evidence for relevance of early urbanization: Traditionally Hippocratic medicine is tied to a single practitioner, Hippocrates of the island of Cos a few miles off the Ionic Coast (now the western coast of Turkey). Reasons for disagreeing with this attribution are presented elsewhere (*The Natural State of Medical Practice*, volume 1, p. 217ff). It is considered probable that what would become Hippocratic medicine originated with development of the ancient Greek city-states. The best candidate is the large and prosperous primary city of Miletos about fifty miles from the island Cos on the mainland of then Ionia. It was founded as a primary city-state about 1050 BC and reached a population of 10,000 by 800 BC. Whatever the conclusions may be about the site of its origin, there is no doubt but that 5th C BC Hippocratic medicine originated during a century or more prior to Hippocrates (his dates supposedly 460-380 BC), for the breadth and depth of its medical knowledge had to have been acquired by many physicians over at least two or three generations and shared collegially. It is in line with this reasoning that the history and prehistory of Miletos is considered the paradigm city where Hippocratic medicine probably began sometime in the 6th C BC, an unprovable opinion because Miletos was razed to the ground by the Persians in 496 BC. There is no evidence of a burgeoning 6th C BC medical practice in any other ancient Greek city-state.

Evidence for authoritarian manipulation: Hippocratic medicine had a short run of productivity. Its disintegration was part of the disintegration of the ancient Greek city-state and its democratic foundations, beginning in the 4th C BC, and completed by the Roman army in 146 BC. Disruption of Greek civilization, like that which followed the Early Dynastic period of Sumer, also disrupted the medical associations that had fostered medical progress. Sadly, the Roman Empire developed no formal medical profession of its own, relying instead on foreign practitioners. As a consequence, when the Dark Ages arrived there were no medical professionals remaining.

Conclusions[24]

For more than a century-and-a-half the West has reaped the benefits of medical progress that began in the 18th C, and it seems unimaginable that present-day benefits could be lost. But the five ancient civilizations identified herein initiated rational medical practices and then lost the benefits of medical progress as centralization of political power disrupted and arrogated the practice of medicine. Our modern medicine also began as a consequence of resurgent autonomy that can be traced to the Reformation (*The Natural*

---

[23] See this website's Section "Papers" for my contributions to date.

[24] For factual support of much of the following see Book IV, volume 1, of *The Natural State of Medical Practice*.

State of Medical Practice, volume 1, p. 458ff). Might centralization of political power in the West lead to the same disruptions for us?

The issue involves the unprivileged population, or common citizenry, to which can be traced all medical progress. In ancient times it was the common practitioner who, acquiring a certain knack or discovering an unusual effect of a botanical, acquired a slight reputation as a local healer. It also was in ancient times that, when the demographic situation was suitable, several such healers decided to share their knowledge so as to improve their services. Over a century, or two, or three, and if social circumstances remained relatively stable, that number increased and their reputation did as well, providing future compilers, collators and editors with the knowledge that would find its way into the medical classics described herein. These early practitioners did not suddenly appear because of royal edict, and there was no template to guide their initial collegial associations. They were merely everyday citizens who, realizing their services were useful to their circle of acquaintances and basing their effort on autonomous self-betterment, decided to improve those services by sharing and critiquing their knowledge and then expanding its delivery to the general population. A profession was born. And that is what a settlement hierarchy permitted during in early urbanization; it provided the opening for a variety of services to spontaneously appear and to freely evolve before political forces came on the scene.

There were the inevitable seemingly miraculous cures, and this would contribute to beliefs in healing deities and medical superpowers. Some of the diagnoses, therapies and prognostics of early healers would be spectacularly correct and such feats elevated the popularity of the medical practitioner. But inevitable as well were similar pronouncements and healing that appeared to be successes of seers and exorcists. Clinical practitioners obviously knew the difference, and thus the earliest expressions of medical practice in Sumer, India, China and ancient Greece appear to have been free of mysticism. And it turned out that, for the time being, the clinical practitioner and the exorcist were not mutually exclusive. Both responded to a social need, and the state of knowledge was not yet so great as to overwhelmingly favor one or the other. They worked in parallel but not in concert.

Then matters changed. With the inevitable centralization of political power in their respective city-states, government favored some types of medical practices politically useful or popular, especially if they reflected some intimate association with the divine. In Sumer the rational *azu* practitioner was diminished by the mystical *asipu* to the point of disappearing altogether for centuries, in Egypt the predynastic community practitioner was incorporated into a pharaonic priesthood, in India the scattered knowledge of earlier Vedic-age clinical practitioners was tied up in the unchanging and mystical wrappings of Hinduism, and in China similar fragments of ancient medical knowledge were compiled by court bibliographers and wrapped in bureaucratic layers of philosophical and therapeutic pseudoscience to accommodate Confucian-oriented political ends. In each case the originators of unvarnished rational medicine have been lost in time, and in each case medical progress either ceased (India, China) or regressed (Mesopotamia, Egypt) rather than progressed.

In ancient Greece the origin of a true medical practice was similar to those in the preceding paragraph, but the combination of a relatively stable social environment and a trend to democratic governance that did not endeavor to interfere with medical services led to the flourish of medical insight documented in the Hippocratic Corpus. It was the authoritarian disruption of the Greek civilization by Philip of Macedon and then Roman armies that provided the colophon to what had been a fruitful beginning.

Medicine in Western civilization began similarly. Arising from the barren medical landscape of the medieval but grandly abetted by the printing press, individual practitioners among the general population began to identify and then communicate features of clinical medicine with their acquaintances. Local practitioners began to replace the medieval university professors of medicine who taught the words but not the methods of the Hippocratics, and, more importantly, to begin their own collegial associations. From these humble practitioners, not the Universities, the Vatican, the Lordships, or Renaissance patronage arose modern medicine. They did not build on previous "shoulders;" they began anew. Slow at first but with astounding successes since the 18th C, the benefits of Western medicine have mollified many of the threats to our health and happiness and, for the first time in human history, increased the life expectancy of a civilization.

That is the story to date. But what now? If there is any lesson to be learned from the history of medical practice as presented in *The Natural State of Medical Practice* it is that its origin and its perpetuation depend on the natural rights and thereby civil liberty of the general population, unleashing its ingenuity and common sense (see Excursus 3). But authoritarian governance of any kind will inevitably attempt to acquire and dominate the services of the medical profession.[25] It will integrate its favored medical practice into a bureaucratic framework for political convenience. The resulting misuse of that medical association will interfere with medical progress. Equally important, *The Natural State of Medical Practice* has disclosed an unintended consequence of that interference, the cessation of the flow of ideas from the general population. The sequestration of medical practice within a privileged political bureaucracy prevents alternative medical insights and inventions from developing. This removal of options for autonomous pursuit of medical care by the unprivileged citizens (in the United States those outside government service or assistance) disenfranchises the ingenuity and common sense of the greater part of society.

There is a lesson to be learned here regarding government intrusion into today's medical practice in the United States, one that in all likelihood can be extended to include other aspects of society. It is not just that medical practice as an arm of a political hierarchy becomes the prerogative of the incompetent, inserts a third party between patient and physician, and, as medicine now belongs in the privileged class, is no longer self-regulated and becomes an invitation for abuse. It is also critical to recognize the great harm done as canonization of governmental medicine marginalizes attempts at improvement from any other source except for those from whom it can also control, *i.e.*, medical corporatism. Alternative ideas become anathema and all that term implies.

It is proper, therefore, to take issue with any inappropriate medical decision by government. But this will inevitably fragment any organized opposition, for there will not be unanimity on many issues. The conclusion of this excursus, therefore, is an appeal

---

[25] To a list of authoritarian governance some might include that pan-European super-kinship, the medieval Church, but it must be understood that true medical practices had disappeared prior to the approach of the Dark Ages. The Church was the only institution that, acting in accord with its moral message, stepped forward to fill that void. The idea that it used its role in medicine to increase its power is untenable. For the most part the Church tried to dissuade a medical component among its adherents. The problem, instead, was lack of autonomy for the common citizenry in feudal Europe, and it is the later interaction between feudal interests and the increasing power of the Church that begot many problems.

to the medical profession to realize the real problem is the forest, not just some of the trees. For medicine, and probably for everything else, that forest is big government.

EXCURSUS 13

An important question regarding the disappearance from five ancient civilizations of early attempts at developing a rational medical profession is why, once they disappeared, there was no further attempt to initiate another. The delayed commencement of modern medicine is a story of enormous consequence, and, after a brief review of the ancient losses, causes of the delay are considered. Two reasons seem most likely, both attributable to an all-powerful political hierarchy: canonization of venerable medical knowledge resistant to change and marginalization of the common citizenry from whom the original rational medical knowledge arose.

CONSEQUENCES AND IMPLICATIONS FOR MEDICINE OF THE MARGINALIZATION OF UNPRIVILEGED MEN AND WOMEN IN ANCIENT CIVILIZATIONS

Introduction

In *The Natural State of Medical Practice* it was shown that, within the great ancient civilizations of Mesopotamia, Egypt, India, China and Greece, early successful efforts at rational/scientific medicine deteriorated as political power centralized.[1] In sympathy with the adage of not seeing the forest for the trees (see opening verse of Excursus 12), root causes are re-examined herein so that we might identify causes for the *permanency* of that deterioration.

This inquiry may also have other ramifications, for historians and philosophers often view the history of civilizations as predictable based on cyclic, linear, economic and other models, some concluding that successive civilizations are in fact gradually progressing over time because of lessons learned from preceding ones. In contrast, *The Natural State of Medical Practice* and the Isagorial Theory of Human Progress it describes provide evidence that human progress, as gauged by medical progress, does not improve in such a fashion. Indeed, with loss of freedom postulated to have existed for the early urban populations of the primary city-states of Mesopotamia, Egypt, India, China and Greece, medical progress *permanently* ceased despite the sequence of prominent and powerful secondary civilizations that followed. It was also observed that following centralization of political power canonization of medicine often seemed to serve as a tool of the political class.[2] Could this persistent inability to progress, which extended over many centuries, even millennia, be explained solely on the loss of freedom?

---

[1] See volume 1 of *The Natural State of Medical Practice*, Book I, chapters 2-6, and Book III, chapters 1-2.

[2] What followed centralization of political power as primary city-states were engulfed within the evolving civilizations of Mesopotamia, Egypt, India and China might be considered either (1) a sequence of authoritarian civilizations or (2) one prolonged civilization with its ups and downs, but medical progress in either case remained at baseline empiricism. This suggests that the entire concept of cycling or other predictable sequences of civilizations may be a phantom of no particular value.

The role of freedom

A prominent modern thinker on freedom was the psychologist, Dr. Mortimer Adler, who postulated three types of freedom of the individual:[3]

1. Social (circumstantial) freedom
2. Psychological freedom (free will)
3. Moral freedom

Now (2) and (3) reflect intrinsic freedoms effected by individual action. But the medical profession affects and is affected by many people and events. Furthermore, medical progress itself was shown, in *The Natural State of Medical Practice*, to be a group function requiring a composite of individual efforts. Many external pressures come to bear on medicine. So present focus is on Adler's social, or circumstantial, freedom, *i.e.*, freedom that varies according to prevailing circumstance.

Issues of social freedom can be even more precisely defined if the focus is on the restriction of choices rather than freedom of the individual to choose from a great variety of available choices. The effect of external constraints on choice is important to determine because it suggests that human progress can be blocked even if civil liberties of the individual are maintained. In other words, even in Western nations that have prospered so upon protection of individual civil liberties (based on natural rights), it would be possible to lose all and, for Western civilization, or any civilization, to cease or roll back medical progress with freedoms seemingly intact (also see graph, *The Natural State of Medical Practice*, volume 1, p. 580).

Historical assessment

What characterized the role played by the ancient governments of Mesopotamia, Egypt, India, China and Greece that led to loss of true medical practitioners and was it actively or passively pursued for centuries? To summarize, two features characterized the role by which institutionalized political power affected the practice of rational medicine in the long term:

1. Mesopotamian monarchical governments placed punitive controls on early Sumerian community practitioners, thus discouraging new entrants into the profession. Akkadian conquerors, in their commercial unification of the Sumerian city-states, appeared to devalue the significance of those practitioners by favoring the palace favorites, exorcists. Despite this, Sumerian medical knowledge, as with Sumerian knowledge in other technical areas, was canonized as superior, and, except for addition of mystical components and chants during subsequent empires, remained little changed even to the 7th C BC. In addition, the role of enforced work, required by the State and elite classes, was widespread and included much more than overt slavery. Monarchical states took over the temples and allocated land and servile populations to select elites, working hand-in-hand

---

[3] M. Adler, *Idea of Freedom*, New York, 1958, pp. xxvii, 689, and Adler and M. Weismann, *How to Think about the Great Ideas: From the Great Books of Western Civilization*, Chicago, 2001, chapter 18.

with their development. Options for commerce and specialization open to the average citizen, seen during the initial urbanization periods of the city-states, were not present under subsequent totalitarian leadership. The possibility of a resurgent and autonomous collegial association of practitioners capable of furthering medical progress would have been remote.[4]

2. In Egypt early community practitioners were integrated into palace hierarchy as priests and made part of its conservative bureaucracy. Two things happened. First, the original medical observations and writings later identified in the *Papyrus Ebers* were canonized. This veneration made them resistant to change. Second, the far greater part of the population worked in specified crafts and trades, usually familial, or were peasants tied to the land. The economy, a system of redistribution, and even wages were determined by the State, and social mobility was difficult. Even though the Egyptian citizenry was, unlike its slaves, free (*e.g.*, the legal autonomy of women was similar to that of men), its predetermined and rigidly regulated economy precluded the option of a spontaneous collegial association of professional practitioners, especially if they might be competition for the priest-physicians.

3. In India there were also two events that prevented medical progress. First, the early Brahminic institutions of Hinduism collected and amended the medical knowledge of an earlier civilization, retaining the original but editing it as the *Charaka Samhita*, thus making their specialized knowledge resistant to change and consistent with the Laws of Manu. Second, over the centuries in a disunited subcontinent, medical guilds appeared in large cities, but these, like Renaissance guilds, were monopolistic institutions protected by the local monarch in return for favors. A competitive medical association capable of progress would not have been permitted. Wandering solitary mendicant practitioners would have been unable to form collegial associations to improve their product.

4. In Chinese dynastic governments select medical practitioners were integrated into an elite medical bureaucracy. There were two consequences in medicine. First, collected original medical observations of a much earlier age were codified in the *Huang Ti Nei Ching Su Wen* and canonized by that medical bureaucracy, thus becoming resistant to change. Second, with the far greater part of the population being poor and servile, options for forming an autonomous medical profession were nonexistent. Wandering individual medical practitioners, the "bell-ringers," could not form medical associations to collegially share and improve their knowledge, instead being at times even competitive with each other, their knowledge unrecorded.

5. In contrast to the preceding civilizations, the Greco-Roman civilization did not canonize Hippocratic medicine, and the option of forming an autonomous collegial profession was not closed to the people. But there still were the same two consequences. First, social disruption caused by wars and conquests discouraged investment in medical careers by the

---

[4] The clever ways by which monarch and oligarch were able to organize and control land and workforce is considered in detail by: Tenney, J. S., *Babylonian Populations, Servility and Cuneiform Records*, in *Journal of the Economic and Social History of the Orient*, 60:715-787, 2017.

average citizen, and Hippocratic medicine gradually disappeared, only to be rediscovered and canonized during the Dark Ages and Medieval Period and thus resistant to change even into the 18th C. Secondly, local political hierarchies in a feudal Europe assigned the far greater part of the population to serfdom with few options for self-betterment.

In the five civilizations under discussion there were two important consequences of governmental misappropriation of existing medical knowledge. One was canonization of the original knowledge, thus making it resistant to improvement. This was not purposely done. Essentially, that original knowledge was canonized as it became venerable over time because there was nothing else with which to replace it. Thus, the primary issue in this excursus does not revolve around the original medical practitioners or their knowledge, although the role of canonization will be more closely examined in a future excursus. The primary issue remains: why was there no replacement.

The second consequence was unanticipated. In four of the five civilizations centralized political governance and a rigidly controlled economy led to marginalization of the general population. Because a medical "profession" had been integrated into the bureaucracies of ancient Sumer, Egypt and China a parallel medical profession arising among the common citizenry was remote. But more importantly, as elite classes increased their regional control, most of the population were relegated to little more than serfdom. The options for self-betterment were limited or nonexistent, collegial associations of medical practitioners did not develop, and medical progress did not occur. In ancient India the situation was different: following the decline of the Indus River Valley city-states no sizeable cities would appear for over a thousand years and individual practitioners were peripatetic, presumably because demographic requirements for a nascent medical profession did not exist. In Greece, Hippocratic medicine vanished because its practitioners were not renewed as ancient Greco-Roman civilization ended. Feudalism then enchained the bulk of the European population for more than a thousand years.

Conclusion

As more completely described in *The Natural State of Medical Practice* (volume 3), it is postulated that the importance of the unprivileged, or common citizenry, in developing rational medical practices in five great civilizations predominated at their founding. In a sense, at that early state of urbanization everyone was relatively "unprivileged." They were the source of practitioners, the source of medical ingenuity, and the source of autonomous associations that included a nascent rational medical profession.

The subsequent appropriation of medical practitioners by early governments as described above was important. But what the present historical assessment brings to attention is the mechanism by which policies of large government can be so destructive for so long. A mere temporary lapse of a credible medical presence for perhaps one or a few generations following integration of practitioners into the political bureaucracy might have been replenished by a subsequent generation of practitioners arising from the general population. Instead, the political hierarchy poisoned the well from which the original medical advances were drawn, namely the unprivileged general citizenry. By control over the entire social environment to pursue objectives of the State, the option of a collegial association of persons with similar goals of self-betterment was closed to the general population. Occupations became familial and devoid of choice.

This was not done by direct command and it was not done for the purpose of abolishing the goal of health improvement. No laws were passed and nothing was directly taken from the general population for the purpose of depriving them of it. Instead, the mere presence of the social environment that resulted from a rigid political hierarchy was to blame.

Seeing that circumstances other than clear-cut legal and targeted transgression of individual freedom were involved in this social calamity, it is appropriate to re-examine freedom of choice, Adler's "social freedom" and its limitation by "circumstances." He does not pursue the consequences of circumstantial limitations on the range of choices. But it is clear they can be monstrous, for it was the limitation on social "circumstances" rather than edicts that prevented a spontaneous reappearance of collegial affiliations of medical practitioners. In the ancient civilizations described herein restrictions by authoritarian governance spanned society. The general population may have retained "freedom of choice" in many daily activities, but the choices of work were profoundly limited. In the hands of technically ignorant authoritarian governments, severe consequences would descend on the general populations of the five civilizations over the next two thousand years.[5] Does this have relevance to modern medicine?

Four out of five great civilizations assessed for their history of medical practice displayed a similar pattern, and our present course seems to be running parallel with them. (India's Indus River Valley civilization had no replacement.) Arising from the 16th C Reformation and appearing in the general population of the 18th C, medical progress in the West has been remarkable as proven by a global increase in human longevity. But in the last century there has been an inexorable increase in the role of government in the practice of medicine in the United States and a concurrent decrease in individual physicians in private practice. The presence of the federal government is felt, directly or indirectly, in many areas, and intrusions into the relation between physician and patient are ubiquitous.

It is unseemly that governments of Western "democratic" nations would purposely take back the power of the people. And they are not taking that power back. But they are more than willing to accept it when offered, and many people in Western democracies are ceding personal decisions and responsibility to their central governments to manage on their behalf and over which they have little control. At the same time, (1) political power is increasingly concentrated in fewer and fewer persons, and (2) inevitably as government grows there is a simultaneous concentration of incompetence, for the fount of competence lies with the unprivileged citizens. The importance of centralized

---

[5] There is powerful philosophical justification for this position. Dr. Adler (see reference 4) noted that "Freedom consists in a man acting as he pleases, being able to do what he wishes, being able to execute, carry out his desire. A man can have this freedom even if his wishes or his desires were themselves determined." He appends the thinking of the eminent 18th C American theologian and philosopher, Jonathan Edwards: "a man is free if he can do as he wishes, even if he cannot wish as he wishes, meaning that I may not be able to determine my own wishes, but if whatever I wish I am able to execute and carry out, then in so far forth, I am free." For Dr. Edwards, a strong proponent of Calvinist predetermination, it is God who determines what one may wish. Thus, government, by limiting options for the general population of society and thereby interfering in what could be wished by the marginalized (and generally impoverished) population, is acting as God.

incompetence cannot be overestimated as a fundamental flaw of centralized governance. It is not lessened by inclusion in government of select consultants with a point of view. There is already a shift in focus in America from the well-being of the individual patient to the well-being of the subjects of the State such as now exists in China, an anathema to the Hippocratic Oath.

What to do? Some suggestions will be offered in Excursus 17. But in general medical practice needs to be solely in the hands of the medical practitioner. We should remember that the purpose of organizing in medicine is to get better, not bigger. The more medicine comes under the aegis of the political class, the more restricted is the physician's approach to the individual patient, fewer are the options in diagnosis and therapy for the patient, and more limited is the opportunity for a new observation, idea or innovation to be validated.[6] There is canonization of medicine reminiscent of the ancient civilizations, although it is more subtle. These are today's issues.

Thus, a big issue for the future of medicine is **choice** rather than **freedom of choice**. It is about the range of options. The more control central government has over society and its industries, professions, and institutions, the fewer will be the choices of those outside of government. As has always happened, it is the progeny and proponents of the "privileged class" who will have the greater options of a career choice. In medicine this will moderate the effect on society for a while. Government regulations on the profession will prefer those applicants deemed politically correct. But for the rest of the citizenry choice be limited. Gradually, progress will be suppressed, despite claims to the contrary. The solution, of course, is to defeat the specter of big government, for greater will be the variety of solutions emerging and the more likely there will be successful ones.

---

[6] At the end of Excursus 17 is appended the contents of the medical journal *Lancet* from early July, 1962, and early July, 2022. In the former there 22 articles and letters to the editor that specifically involved clinical care; in the latter there was 1. For the *New England Journal of Medicine* from the same dates the difference is less stark but limited to "articles:" 5 from the 1962 date and 2 from the 2022 date, with a third being a report of the first genetically modified porcine-to-human cardiac transplantation, the patient dying a month later.

EXCURSUS 14

In this excursus the novel declaration is made and argued that our present "Western" civilization is the only true civilization in human history.

CIVILIZATION VS. UNCIVILIZATION[1]

"Not only the individual advances from infancy to manhood but the species itself from rudeness to civilization." [2]

Adam Ferguson (1723-1816)

Introduction

It is more than disturbing to read daily the homages to great civilizations inevitably mentioned in most things historical. The idea that we are required to attribute our present achievements and good fortune to some form of ancient greatness is, I suppose, an attempt to appear to be fair, just as is our attempt to blame our own shortcomings on historical events that have prevented our own greatness from becoming manifest. Great men, great empires, and great civilizations seem to provide convenient physical and moral explanations for present-day successes and failures.

The Natural State of Medical Practice introduced a quite different dynamic:

(1) First, it presented objective evidence that Western civilization owes nothing whatever to any other preceding or contemporary civilization other than its necessary genetic makeup.

(2) Second, it refutes the "great man" theory of progress by presenting evidence that genius is widely and equally distributed throughout every society, from which the inarguable conclusion is that it is some society-wide feature that inhibits the manifestation of that genius, not the individual genius.

(3) Third, it identifies all the "great" civilizations as not at all great, instead each being a series of authoritarian/totalitarian regimes that are tacked together to form some sort of geographically connected pseudo-civilization that should be a source of embarrassment rather than a source of pride, civilizations that we would prefer to think have endured because of logic and genius rather than the true cause, barbaric wars to enlarge their desirable geography and extract wealth and power from others.

---

[1] Volume and page number of otherwise unreferenced statements in this monograph refer to the version of the three volumes of *The Natural State of Medical Practice* as published by Liberty Hill Press in 2019:

Vol. 1 – *The Natural State of Medical Practice: An Isagorial Theory of Human Progress*
Vol. 2 – *The Natural State of Medical Practice: Hippocratic Evidence*
Vol. 3 - *The Natural State of Medical Practice: Escape from Egalitarianism*

[2] Adam Ferguson, *An Essay on the History of Civil Society*, London, 1767, beginning of Section I.

(4) And lastly, "great civilizations" are shown to inevitably revert to a primitive empiricism as they age rather than being a steppingstone to the next and better civilization.

The Natural State of Medical Practice concludes, based on the Isagorial Theory of Human Progress derived from it, that the origin of a civilization is commercial enterprise around which city-states evolve. It then arrives at "civilization" status when, working together, it has developed specializations, such as medical professionals, previously unknown to the people, and benefits become available to all. It is progressing and is now "civilized." Then, in a few locations in history, these embryonic "civilizations" coalesced, covering larger regions. I refer here to primary civilizations: predynastic and early dynastic Sumer, predynastic Egypt, the Indus River Valley civilization, the Longshan culture of China, and archaic Greece.[3] Sadly, civilizing ceases at the point when authoritarian political hierarchies achieve ascendancy and supplant the primary ones. Histories of the regions are thereafter characterized by sequential totalitarian regimes that might be likened to economic "bubbles" but are far more tragic. Historians often refer to those sequential secondary civilizations as "great" because of vast regional domination: Mesopotamian, Egyptian, Chinese and Greco-Roman. The Indus River Valley primary civilization is exempt from this charge because its disappearance in history was probably related to geo-climatic change rather than being engulfed by its secondary civilization.

This excursus is meant to crystallize the preceding evidence and to clarify the definition of "civilization." It will then claim at its conclusion that, after several failed attempts at progress, it is our own civilization, commonly identified as "Western," that is the only true civilization, that all other "civilizations" have been the bane of progress and therefore undeserving of the title, and that we are in great danger of following in their footsteps.

Definition

Nationalization means the process of becoming nationalized; ionization means the process of becoming ionized; civilization, therefore, means the process of becoming civilized, and to be civilized, according to Merriam-Webster, is to show "an advanced stage of social and cultural development." This definition, by its use of "social" and the quotation that begins this excursus, means "civilized" should encompass all citizens of a civilization, in contrast to the uncivilized, who remain rude and barbaric.[4]

The present definitions imply an intrinsic superiority of civilization over no civilization. But is that appropriate? Was the Aztec civilization, which was based on

---

[3] A primary civilization is one that has not been "shaped by substantial dependence on or control by other, more complex societies." See: Trigger, B. G., *Understanding Early Civilizations,* Cambridge (UK), 2003, p. 19.

[4] The term "civilization" as used today is relatively new. In Samuel Johnson's 1755 Dictionary of the English Language it is defined as "a law, act of justice, or judgment, which renders a criminal process civil," *i.e.,* its use was legalistic. The word is not even included in his octavo edition of 1760. But notably he references John Locke's use of the word "civilized:" "Amongst those who are counted the civilized part of mankind, this original law of nature still takes place." He is referring to natural law and he applies it to all persons in a civilization, not just a sub-population.

military conquest in part to acquire captives for its vast human sacrifices, superior or culturally advanced over primitive and uncivilized sedentary, horticultural and herding societies? Inhumanity exists in any society, but bigger is surely no guarantor of better, and is usually the opposite: the bigger the pack, the meaner the dog.

With the preceding as a starting point, it might be asked if it is appropriate to speak of any past civilization in glowing terms. I would answer, it is not. Referring to the five "great" civilizations that are examined in *The Natural State of Medical Practice*, the argument is that, in general terms, a bipartite division of citizens existed in each of those civilizations: one segment, the politically powerful elite, included those refined in culture but barbaric in action, and the other segment, vastly larger, included those rude in acculturation but restrained in action. To truly qualify for status as a civilization, I propose the citizenry at large should generally show cultural appreciation and restraint and should not be rude and barbaric in action. The five "great" civilizations to be discussed in this analysis are therefore not entitled to use the term "civilization." In a word, no rigidly authoritarian society is entitled to be a civilization, just as Frederick Douglass stated there can be no virtue without freedom.[5]

Given the tradition surrounding the use of "civilization" over the past three centuries, it can be argued that my rhetorical excess in the preceding is, for all practical purposes, meaningless. But consider the following:

a. The history of China from the Shang Dynasty (1600-1046 BC) to Qing Dynasty (1636-1912) is a sequence, over 3500 years, of more than seventy major kinship-based authoritarian dynasties that ruled, serially or in parallel, *without exception*, by force and conquest. Museums globally display magnificent works of artistry, usually characteristic of a particular dynasty, but the term "civilization" can barely be applied to the region. The elite class, or dynastic kinship, was, overall, ruthless and barbaric in its penchant for war and domination of others, whereas the ninety percent of the population that was the source of the plenty that made possible the tastefulness of the ruling class was poor, fettered and unlettered.

b. The ancient Egyptian civilization historically spans roughly 3500 BC to 525 BC, and encompasses, over those 3000 years, twenty-six dynastic periods of rigid authoritarian rule plagued by internal and external wars, probably owing its long existence primarily to the fact that on the west it was protected by a vast desert and on the east by the Red Sea. We marvel at its art, temples and pyramids, but all this was done on the backs of a servile population and enslaved conquered peoples. Again, the ruling class was conservatively tasteful in its art and architecture but barbaric in its wars and in its domination of captives, slaves, and the general populace. The common people were malnourished, exploited and manipulated.

c. Ancient Mesopotamian city-state dynasties began in Sumer *ca.* 2900 BC but then were forcibly unified by the Akkadians in 2350 BC, passing through the hands of a variety of conquerors and remaining rigidly totalitarian for 4,000 years to include the Persian Empire. Several periods were notable for their art,

---

[5] Foner, P. S., editor, *The Life and Writings of Frederick Douglass*, New York, 1950, in 5 vols., vol. 2, pp. 182-183. With a broader compass D. D'Souza wrote: "Without freedom there is no virtue: A coerced virtue is no virtue at all." See his *Letters to a Young Conservative*, New York, 2002, p. 16. I realize, of course, that there are degrees of authoritarianism. In this excursus "authoritarian" means exceedingly authoritarian.

architecture and scholarship, but it was the ruthless elite and militant classes that shaped the cultural accomplishments of that region, not the illiterate citizenry who were the source of its food and its foot-soldiers.

d. The story is different in ancient India in that its earliest "civilization," that of the Indus River Valley (flourished 2500-2000 BC), appears to have been throughout much of its existence a relatively egalitarian one, in that a hierarchy of dominating political power seems not to have existed. Unless more evidence to the contrary is obtained, it may truly be considered to have been a "civilization," although its duration was cut short by geo-climatic change. What followed was a widely scattered system of monarchies, dynasties and empires down through the Mughal empire (1526-1857) that saw the arrival of colonial powers. These were mostly absolute monarchies characterized by incessant wars, and their empires cannot be considered civilizations. In those few dominions overseen by enlightened leaders, both the monarchical nature of governance and the caste system of social organization maintained a large subject population with limited choice. Hindu Chola art and Islamic Mughal art represent the culture of elite classes that were barbaric in their social controls and conquests, the Chola Dynasty (850-1279) through some thirty rulers and the Mughal Empire (1526-1757) with twenty. Combining regional authoritarian empires or dynasties under a single rubric is a fabrication, not a civilization.

e. Greco-Roman "civilization" also was consumed with wars of conquest. Greek democracies of various types were instituted for the first time in the 6th C BC, and concurrently art, literature, architecture and specializations such as medical practice flourished at all levels of society. The beginnings of a true civilization were apparent and were bearing fruit. But as time passed oligarchical political power and the occasional totalitarian regained prominence and the increased opportunity that had existed for the average citizen was oriented toward preservation of the State (for which their participation was actively sought) rather than self-betterment. Macedonian and Roman conquests ended it all. Even the Pax Romana included wars, particularly the horrors of the Jewish-Roman wars, and a doubling of the area of Roman domination, with the Roman and Romanized elite maintaining a firm hold on plebeian and slave populations.

If a civilization does not somehow identify with the word "civilized," then perhaps some other term should be used to describe the long sequences of serial despotic rule that characterize most human cultures, thereby reserving the term "civilization" for the true thing. When discussing Arnold Toynbee's inevitable cycling of twenty-one civilizations, perhaps we should not be including true civilizations among the doomed, for in his theory there is an implication that all civilizations carry within themselves the seeds of inherent destruction. This excursus proposes that true civilizations do not, that the durability of a "free" civilization has yet to be determined, that nevertheless serious internal dangers exist, and that we in the West had better realize the uniqueness and greatness of our own civilization above all others that have existed lest we throw it away and follow suit.

I would highlight a particular facet of the definition of civilization that will help clarify the significance of the word that some definitions imply, and that is the necessity of objective evidence of *progress*. Progress in the present sense is characterized by purposeful improvement over an existing state of something that benefits members of the civilization. In other words, civilization advances on purpose by seeking utility in ways that benefit all its members, in contrast to culture, which does not change according to any particular goal or plan, and to a dynasty, which exists to benefit the kinship. As discussed in *The Natural State of Medical Practice* (volume 3, p. 211*ff*), a key gauge of progress in a society is its medical care, and an objective measure of effectiveness of that care is life expectancy. Applying this to the "great civilizations" that value was found to be little more than thirty years for the average men and women who made up the great majority of their populations, the same as reported for Stone Age humans and even Neanderthals.[6] Only our own civilization has a claim to human longevity, and even that has been late in coming (see Excursus 9).

It is noteworthy that within this critique of the definition of civilization there is in our modern Western civilization no formal ruler such as is implied in "dynasty" and "empire." Occasionally a ruler might transiently pop up, a Napoleon, Hitler, or Mussolini, only to be snuffed out, by force when necessary, thus preventing the extreme centralization of political power historically represented by Rome, Babylon, Moscow and Beijing.

To conclude, the proposed definition of "civilization" is minimally changed from volume 1, p. 21, of *The Natural State of Medical Practice*:

> "An autonomous urban and rural population sufficiently large to require a regulatory hierarchy to optimize production of a food surplus and trade that contributes to wealth and permits specialization of crafts and vocations capable of progress to the benefit of all citizens."

To cycle or not to cycle

There have been many theories to explain the passage of civilizations, the two most often discussed being cycling and a linear religious unfolding, the former proposed as an explanation for the course of history, each civilization passing through successive phases and ultimately being deposed.

Two 20th C analyses of civilization that have been particularly popular were proposed by Dr. Will Durant and his wife, Ariel, in *The Story of Civilization*, and Dr. Arnold Toynbee in *A Study of History*.[7] The Durants asked, in their *The Lessons of History*, if human progress was real. They noted that "... progress in science and technique has involved some tincture of evil and good," that "we frolic in our emancipation from theology" but have we developed a "natural ethic?," and in scholarly debate it is not clear who would win the "prize," the ancients or the moderns.[8] They concluded by equating progress with heritage. The history of our civilization, with its "saints, statesmen, ...poets, artists...lovers, and philosophers," has provided us with a human heritage of great richness that increases over time and makes our lives fuller. There seems, therefore, to have been hesitancy in acknowledging both the reality and the value of human progress, from which one might conclude that no qualitative distinction exists among the various civilizations, quite a remarkable opinion of their own time. They

---

[6] Bocquet-Appel, J., and Degioanni, A., *Neanderthal Demographic Estimates,* in *Current Anthropology*, 54:S202- S213, 2013.

[7] Will and Ariel Durant, *The Story of Civilization*, New York, 1935-1975, in eleven volumes. Arnold Toynbee, *A Study of History*, London, 1934-1961, in twelve volumes.

[8] Will and Ariel Durant, *The Lessons of History*, New York, 1968, chapter 13.

did acknowledge, however, that "History repeats itself, but only in outline and in the large" (*op. cit.*, p. 88).

Dr. Toynbee approached the history of civilizations differently, writing of the cycling of civilizations in his memorable work, *A Study of History*. He considered a civilization to have started in the response of a local culture to a regional challenge that the great civilizations have overcome by inventing and adapting successfully, the others perishing. Once successful, they grow and prosper as long as they manage new challenges. They fade when their ability to adapt is lost, and it is lost because centralized power fails to meet a challenge, upon which the mass of the population gets upset and then attempts to obtain control. But a rigidly authoritarian resistance is then expanded by the politically powerful, stifling creativity and adaptability. The end has arrived.

I mention the Durants' and Toynbee's theories as paradigmatic, two among many, for most theories of civilizations are enigmatic, and the purpose of this excursus is to present quite a different paradigm.[9]

But consider first another way of looking at cycling of civilizations, namely that it is not civilizations that have cycled. Rather, there is a cycling within each of the many authoritarian dynasties encompassed within a regional culture.[10] Technically the history of each dynasty would be little more than a military history rather than a social one. These strings of authoritarian dynasties might be likened to strings of economic bubbles in their flourishing and collapse. With an apology for repetition, here is a summary:

(a) The Chinese "civilization" can be viewed as merely a prolonged sequence of some seventy serial and overlapping major authoritarian dynasties, each with kinship as its basis, coercion as its method, and an average duration of about one hundred years.

(b) The history of Egypt is similar; a sequence of twenty-six dynasties, some familial, some being conquests, but each with its ruler or sequence of rulers. Egypt had, of course, a governmental bureaucracy that no civilization would ever match, one attended by a myriad of priests that felt the pulse (metaphorically) of the kingdom and provided a conservative regulatory coterie of civil servants that served stabilization and durability for two millennia despite military adventures and misadventures.

(c) Mesopotamian dynasties comprise the history of late Sumerian city-states, the Akkadian empire, a dynastic sequence of Amorite rulers related to Hammurabi, followed by Kassite, Hittite, Neo-Babylonian, Assyrian, Persian and other dynasties. Although these were often not familial, all were militaristic.

To read the histories of Mesopotamian, Egyptian and Chinese "civilizations" is to read of perpetual authoritarian wars and intrigues. The cycling of these supposed civilizations I propose to be an inevitable consequence of authoritarian government that resulted in the *recycling* of pseudo-civilizations as they continuously play at "king of the

---

[9] But Oswald Spengler (1880-1936) should be mentioned here. He proposed *cultural* cycling with the final stage being civilization itself, predicting a century ago the end of our Western culture. Culture, based on his philosophical theory of history, can be likened to an organism with a predictable course and span of life, the reasons supporting his metaphor not given. Spengler's theory and prediction will gain support if our civilization continues in its authoritarian ways, for, as civilization is the final stage in Spengler's definition of culture, we are already living in that stage and it will soon fail if he predicted correctly.

[10] As an example, a local strong man becomes a military leader, conquers the regional army, and becomes king. He is succeeded by his son who conquers a neighboring region to the east and passes the larger kingdom to his three sons. One of the sons poisons the other two and is declared king. After putting down a farmers' rebellion, his weakened forces are overcome by an army from the neighboring region to the west, and the dynasty ends with the king's beheading.

mountain." The only civilized people, when they have not been required to man an army, seem to have been the common citizenry, the unprivileged folk living in scattered poor villages even in today's totalitarian states. As a general statement regarding societies, I think most travelers would agree that the kindest people are the poorest, despite having little to share.

India, as previously stated, was different in that at least some of the initial city-states of the Indus River Valley "civilization" of 2500-2000 BC do not reveal evidence of dynastic, monarchical, or centralized political control.

Our admiration of civilizations is usually expressed in our opinions of their culture, their arts, their discoveries and the individuals associated with these. We may even admire powerful and large dynasties because of their military "genius" and conquests. But what we traditionally call "civilizations" are judged on the basis of their cultural achievements, not their civility. This is like admiring lipstick on a pig and should change.

To conclude, it has yet to be determined if true civilizations have an intrinsic cycle. True civilizations have been few and short-lived because of their displacement by political hierarchies of power. But it is noteworthy that some of their initial accomplishments have been remembered throughout the duration of subsequent authoritarian cycling dynasties. For example, writing and medical legacies (*i.e.*, the ancient medical classics) associated with transient nascent true civilizations apparently do not cycle. They tend to be retained even when subsequent authoritarian dynasties have been unable to build on them.

Enter natural law

In *The Natural State of Medical Practice* and in Excursus 6 the concept of natural law is considered in detail and its expression in the ethical component of the Ten Commandments and in the Golden Rule as protecting our natural rights is described. The equivalent of natural law has found expression in most cultures in which it has been sought; it can also be considered one's conscience. We have, therefore, a general concurrence as to the reality of natural law and an approximate agreement on its content, even though there are varying opinions on its source.

Natural law protects our natural rights from infringement by others. It is logical that this protection should include institutional infringements, including those from government. It was propounded in *The Natural State of Medical Practice* that human progress is a natural consequence of protection of natural rights, at least if we use medical practice as a gauge. It proposes as well that a society that does not abide by natural law and thereby denies natural rights will not progress.

Now translate the preceding into a political system. The difference between authoritarian and nonauthoritarian governance is that in a free society a person acquires wealth, and in sense power, by providing a desired product. It is a system of popular exchange, a mutual give and take. In contrast, an authoritarian system (socialism, communism, fascism, totalitarianism) does not abide by natural law and punitively takes wealth and power from part or all of the people and uses it for goals of the political hierarchy. Thus, authoritarianism, which also limits the choices of its subjects to exploit self-interest (see Excursus 13), is not just a matter of forcing people to do something they would otherwise not do and limiting what they can do; it is also a matter of taking from people what they would otherwise not give. In a free society the acquisition of power via enterprise is inherently limited by competition; in authoritarian governance there is no limit to acquisition of power. In effect, a free society replaces armored medieval knights serving the local lord with self-serving but humane merchants who respect the rights of others.

Thus, to those who have lived in a free society, authoritarianism seems a bad idea, whether in its abuse of power or in its acquisition of power. And so it is sad today that many people are surrendering their rights and responsibilities to central government, for by doing these things authoritarian persons and groups quickly acquire power at no personal cost or effort; authoritarianism is being readily abetted rather than resisted. Active accretion of power is an inevitable accompaniment of any authoritarian system, and it inevitably concentrates that power in the hands of fewer and fewer persons.

From this perspective, authoritarianism cannot be seen as ever doing good, and any apparent good it seems to do is merely camouflage for casting a net to acquire more followers and thus have more power. A related goal of authoritarian process is to obviate any other source of power that might pose a threat. Contradictory ideas are prevented from being heard. In Mao Zedong's China, the purpose of government was not to enforce equity; it was to make people the same and so be rid of opposition by defining and indoctrinating what a citizen must be and do.

As for making people the same, this is not possible, and therefore authoritarianism is characterized by wars in perpetuity. And if that were not enough, (1) to enforce equity will cause human progress to promptly cease, and (2) the inevitable centralization of incompetence will invite unnatural disasters.

The immorality of authoritarian governance is clear: it offends natural law. It takes things from the people which they do not want to give; it makes people do things they know they shouldn't do; it limits the choices of things they should do; it places man-made laws above natural law; and in doing so it arrogates to itself the right to define good and bad. It is no wonder why it is so terrible. What is a wonder is why people, when they have a choice, would purposely choose it or encourage it.

In prior excursus three important points were made:
(1) The ethical commandments of the Decalogue, the Golden Rule and natural law are considered equivalents.
(2) Their application over many centuries has been directed at the individual, not institutions.
(3) By ignoring their institutional significance, natural rights have been transgressed, common men and women over the ages have been denied free expression of their ingenuity, and in doing so human progress has been delayed for millennia.

The immorality that authoritarian government inflicts on the unprivileged majority is an immorality of unimaginable proportions. Centralization of political power must be fervently opposed. We can see from the preceding that empires and dynasties have rulers. In contrast, as described in *The Natural State of Medical Practice* and in the above definition of "civilization," the primary city-states of Sumer, Egypt, India, China and ancient Greece first had *settlement hierarchies* rather than rulers to guide their early development. [11] Analogously, the remarkable successes of our own civilization evolved

---

[11] Definition of a "settlement hierarchy:" "A natural progression of intergroup adjustments that spontaneously occurs as an urbanizing society, having no prior experience with a political hierarchy, becomes more complex and acquires facilities, goods, and services to accommodate an enlarging population." (Volume 3, p. 22, of *The Natural State of Medical Practice*.) The relevance of

at the same time its nations ridded themselves of totalitarian rulers and were adopting popular assemblies. **An essential difference therefore is the absence of consolidated authoritarian rule in a true civilization.**

Civilizations without rulers

Professor Toynbee was able to fill twelve large volumes with his commentary on twenty-one civilizations because their peculiarities abound. But those peculiarities reflect the respective cultures, whereas their houses of power are similar, authoritarians all: kings, pharaohs, monarchs, czars, emperors, tyrants, sultans, kaisers, dictators, fuhrers, etc. In any new magisterial tome on civilizations perhaps there need be but two types of civilizations: authoritarian and nonauthoritarian.

Toynbee also lays the sad course of civilizations on leadership that becomes progressively more authoritarian to the point that innovation and adaptability are lost. There are few who would disagree with that. The problem with any leadership is that the greater the concentration of power the greater is the concentration of incompetence, for the problems of a large civilization are vast and their solutions are to be found among the people of the civilization, not a single or a few individuals.[12] Of great benefit to our nation has been its extraordinary distribution of decision-making throughout society, rather than confining it to a singular locus. This is the essence of Tocqueville's paragraph regarding associations in America that opens Excursus 15: *Progress: Our Most Important Product.*

To summarize the present argument, only one true civilization is recognized today, our own. All other true civilizations were not permitted to survive and grow; they were aborted. Of Dr. Toynbee's list, the Babylonian, Assyrian, Persian, Pharaonic, Chinese and Roman dynasties do not represent civilizations. All instead represent serial authoritarian "bubbles" that burst upon contact with a superior authoritarian "bubble." If it is argued that we in the West have had our share of dynasties, this is not denied, but the difference is that, like whack-a-mole, the authoritarian with an eye for the main chance just pops up here and there rather than being all-consuming, for when they appear the protectors of natural rights have suppressed them. It is through such Western loopholes in authoritarian governance that have developed since the Reformation that natural rights and natural law have gained a commanding foothold, so far.

---

settlement hierarchy as a natural step in early urbanization is strengthened by the positive correlation between organizational complexity and demographic scale (level of tiered hierarchy and population size). See: Sandeford, D. S., 2018, *Organizational Complexity and Demographic Scale in Primary States*, in *R. Soc open sci. 5:171137.http://dx.doi.org/10.1098/rsos.171137*. The text also includes an overview of specific primary "states" in ancient Mesopotamia, Egypt, India and China.

[12] In the same sense, it is arguable that university professors are not, and should not be expected to be, the source of ideas more than any other group. Good ideas emerge from all the people. The professors, appropriately through their studies and writings, provide the intellectual arguments about, for, and against those ideas, enlighten their students on the range of criticism of the subject, and in the process educate them on the importance of critical thinking so that they become discerning in forming their own opinions rather than blindly following the opinions of others, and thereby contribute to the pool of ideas from which progress will continue.

Conclusion: Uncivil civilizations

Civilization is too polite a term for what it is traditionally meant to describe. But there is no word that is a satisfactory alternative to "civilization" just as there is no acceptable antonym. It will remain in use, although hopefully with acceptable qualifications. As for our own civilization, a name for it will be the subject of Excursus 16.

But we must wonder about a future "clash of civilizations." This was the title of a 1996 book by Dr. Samuel Huntington in which he divided the globe among eight contemporary civilizations.[13] The "clash" was not postulated to result from ideology because it seemed apparent to Dr. Huntington that Western technology and democratic freedoms were being accepted and gradually implemented globally. Instead, it would be cultural enmity that sparked conflict. But if our own civilization indeed captures imaginations worldwide and its benefits are globally realized, why would any reasonable person want to destroy that which has improved the lives of so many, an ideology that is both historically successful and spreads because of its beneficence, not its army. True civilizations, in contrast to cultures, should not clash.

To explain this inconsistency the role of the authoritarian again asserts itself. Islam, Orthodox Christianity, Hindu, Buddhist and Shinto, whether viewed as religions or as cultures, have historically been associated with authoritarian regimes, sometimes, as in the West, as a State religion. But the theological message of all these religions includes a desire for peace. While religious support of authoritarian national or dynastic objectives has at times been sought by the politically powerful, it is today only Islam that extensively and intrinsically provides guidance for State action, although regionally this has occurred with all the other religions in the past. I propose that it is not culture, as expressed through dominant religions, that would originate any clash. It would instead emerge from the centralized political power that guides the respective regions encompassing those religions. Of course, there will be attempts to rally religions and other types of cultural support for authoritarian purposes, but behind it all the small number of persons who maintain total political control over the several regions of the globe will be the authors of violence, not the common citizens. For the moment, persons with supreme power reside in Moscow, Pyongyang, Beijing, and Teheran, not in basilicas, temples, shrines and mosques. Furthermore, three of those four centers of political power are, or have been, declared atheistic. Religions, and thereby cultures, are not the issue, and as an example of human variation they are to be valued.

Although modern culture itself therefore seems an unlikely basis for a call to arms, the same cannot be said for authoritarian concentration of power. That is where the risk lies. Our own civilization's demotion of authoritarianism and promotion of natural rights protection has been the key to its success, and this is particularly so for the United States of America and its Constitution. As Ayn Rand wrote in 1982: "I can say – not as a patriotic bromide, but with full knowledge of the necessary metaphysical, epistemological, ethical, political and esthetic roots – that the United States of America is the greatest, the noblest and, in its original founding principles, the only moral country in

---

[13] Samuel P. Huntington, *The Clash of Civilization and the Remaking of World Order*, New York, 1996.

the history of the world."[14] And within our civilization, to equate the United States with any other nation *or attempt to render it so* is an apostasy. But, based on historical evidence of a society's almost irresistible acquiescence over time to concentration of political power and on recent trends to tribalism and restriction of natural rights in the United States, the probability is rising that ours will follow. Huntington's "clash of civilizations" will not be remote if the only true civilization, our own, loses its most potent defender, the United States of America, should we continue to depreciate into just another authoritarian nation.

Rejection of natural law, the authoritarian's procedural guide throughout the ages, will have inescapable consequences, and, as discussed in Excursus 3, its innocent victims will be our descendants.

---

[16] This statement is from the opening essay of Ayn Rand's posthumous book of essays, *Philosophy: Who Needs It?*, Indianapolis, 1982.

EXCURSUS 15

Human progress, which Excursus 14 argued is a necessary component of the definition of a civilization, was proposed in *The Natural State of Medical Practice* to emerge in early societies from individuals collaborating in common council to improve their condition in life. Through such collaborative groups ideas can be improved and vetted to the benefit of the members and, when applied to society, can lead to improvement in the lives of everyone. Thus, whenever the government restricts the natural exploitation of ingenuity for self-betterment, government not only limits an individual's options for his or her personal well-being. It also blocks the benefits that can emerge from a new idea or discovery being introduced into society. Also in this excursus, human ingenuity (as a facet of human reason) is postulated as a counterpart to natural law. Natural law is our protection against other humans, but ingenuity is our protection against everything else. I propose that purposeful limitations by government on one's attempt at improving, by legal means, one's condition in life can be considered equivalent to violation of natural law. It is detrimental to both the individual and society, even to its survival.

PROGRESS: OUR MOST IMPORTANT PRODUCT[1]

> **Nothing, in my opinion, is more deserving of our attention than the intellectual and moral associations of America. The political and industrial associations of that country strike us forcibly; but the others elude our observation, or if we discover them we understand them imperfectly, because we have hardly ever seen anything of the kind. It must, however, be acknowledged that they are as necessary to the American people as the former, and perhaps more so. *In democratic countries the science of association is the mother of science; the progress of all the rest depends upon the progress it has made.*[2] Amongst the laws which rule human societies there is one which seems to be more precise and clearer than all others. If men are to remain civilized, or to become so, the art of associating together must grow and improve in the same ratio in which the equality of conditions is increased.**
> **Alexis de Tocqueville (1805-1859)[3]**

---

[1] Volume and page number of otherwise unreferenced statements in this monograph refer to the version of the three volumes of *The Natural State of Medical Practice* as published by Liberty Hill Press in 2019:
Vol. 1 – *The Natural State of Medical Practice: An Isagorial Theory of Human Progress*
Vol. 2 – *The Natural State of Medical Practice: Hippocratic Evidence*
Vol. 3 - *The Natural State of Medical Practice: Escape from Egalitarianism*
[2] Dans les pays democratiques, la science de l'association est la science-mere; le progres de toutes les autres depend des progres de celle-la. The translation is accurate.
[3] *Democracy in America*, vol. II, sect. 2, chap. 5, (translation of final paragraphs by Henry Reeve, italics added). The referenced chapter by Tocqueville comprehends all types of associations. There is a tendency in academia to exclusively concentrate on his use of associations as bases for activism in the public or "civil" sphere. I view this as a narrow interpretation. Implicit in his overall assessment of associations is self-governance. Management of local issues by local people decouples them from central government: the more widespread the associations the less governmental presence and the less risk of tyranny. To this I would also add is his implication, in the italicized line, that associations are *the mother of science* in that they include those associations

Introduction

In Excursus 14 the definition of "civilization" was contemplated, and it was concluded that there has been only one mature civilization worthy of the name, our own. The unsuccessful candidates included the sequential regional authoritarian governments in ancient Mesopotamia, Egypt, India, China and circum-Mediterranean. But it was also noted that in a primary city-state of each region there was an early period of *progress*, one manifestation of which was medical competence as shown in their ancient medical writings such as exist today. Although some evidence for this conclusion is circumstantial, it points to a period of interest called the "settlement hierarchy." A settlement hierarchy is an early phase of urbanization that has yet to encounter a controlling political hierarchy.[4] But once a centralized political hierarchy supervened, there was cessation of medical progress. For this reason, in Excursus 14 the subsequent authoritarian/totalitarian dynasties and empires that followed on those initial, or "primary," city-states were removed from the social category of "civilization."

On leaving the tribe or clan and entering early urbanization, the developmental stages for progression of a society to the status of "civilization" are:

basic ingenuity > competency > collaboration > invention > civilization
(the individual   **(the associations of the**   **(entire society**
in the tribe)   **settlement hierarchy)**   **benefits)**

The settlement hierarchy represents the collaborative (group or association) phase of urbanization. This excursus examines in greater detail the role of collaboration in generating progress and those factors uncovered by *The Natural State of Medical Practice* that inhibit progress and therefore interfere with the civilizing of society. It will suggest that America has passed through the equivalent of the settlement hierarchy phase (the phase tolerating Tocqueville's "science of association") with its benefits to the entire society and is now encountering a "controlling political hierarchy" and all that entails.

The mechanism of progress: A two-pronged explanation

As stated by Tocqueville in the opening quotation, **the science of association is the mother of science.** It is not enough to merely discover or invent something potentially useful. That has been going on since the first man and woman. It is, instead, the proliferation of that useful discovery or invention throughout one's society that determines its significance and the confirmation and manipulation of that discovery or

---

that encourage, vet and display the ingenuity and inventiveness of the people, the essence of this excursus.

[4] The basis for this proposed explanation is that careful objective studies not only confirm the concept of an early productive growth phase of primary urbanization but also find their structure mathematically predictable in that the complexity of their organizational and regulatory hierarchies correlates with population size. This suggests that all primary city-states or early urban centers experienced, or were capable of experiencing, an initial period of relative freedom from authoritarian control that led to population growth, prosperity and nascent civilization status during the settlement hierarchy stage. See: Sandeford, D. S., *Organizational Complexity and Demographic Scale in Primary States*, in *R. Soc. Open sci.* 5:171137.http://dx.doi.org/10.1098/rsos.171137, 2018.

invention that makes it scientific. In previous ages this required a group effort, for this engaged the ingenuity of several minds to a single purpose, represented a broader platform from which to announce the event, increased the likelihood that any benefit would accrue community-wide, and made it less likely to be ignored, minimized, or scuttled by those in positions of authority.[5]

The populations in the primary city-states of Sumer, Egypt, India, China and ancient Greece were not large by modern standards, and it was proposed that a small group, perhaps but three or four people, might have been sufficient to create a focus of competency in some trade, craft, or service that would grow in membership, improve its product or service and become a popular profession.[6] Logically it follows that a larger group should have more and perhaps better ideas on which to build.

Unfortunately, as population increased this did not happen. Instead, central political hierarchies evolved that would have their own idea about what those better ideas would be, and authoritarian regulation stifled innovation and discovery by the common citizenry. The story of *The Natural State of Medical Practice* is the story of the disastrous consequences resulting from the terribly imperfect competence of authoritarian leadership neglecting the pervasive competence of the people.

America evolved differently. During and after the confluence of the counterpart of "city-states" into a Union, many voluntary associations developed, composed of like-minded people who wanted to improve their personal status, *e.g.*, granges, guilds, lodges, boards, business groups. In contrast to all other contemporary nations, the newly formed government of the United States did not subsequently commandeer sources of power and success from the unifying States; its new Constitution prevented such meddling. This left local problems in the hands of local populations, and local associations appeared that managed, invented, and discovered as their situations required. Their prominence, success, and importance in resisting centralization of power in central government was considered by Tocqueville to surpass that of even "political and industrial associations." Competency, therefore, remained diffusely distributed throughout the land, active and vocal throughout the citizenry, and the inherent limited competency of central government had less opportunity for display. This two-pronged approach of (1) personal autonomy and (2) limited government led to the many successes of our society and to its progress, producing the greatest nation in the history of the world.[7]

A group discussion

"Groups" as a concept in the modern social sciences has received much attention, especially "primary" groups "characterized by intimate face-to-face association and cooperation." [8] Primary groups have been further divided into (1) those of common blood

---

[5] Modern communication, digital technology and ready access to capital make individual entrepreneurs less dependent on collegial associations to devise, develop, and widely distribute a discovery or invention.

[6] This is proposed in *The Natural State of Medical Practice*, vol. 1, p. 168*ff*, in the excursus describing the ancient Greek association called a "koinon."

[7] While the focus herein is mostly the United States of America, the political relevance of natural rights and natural law originated in Europe following the Reformation. See volume 1, p. 439*ff*.

[8] Charles H. Cooley, *Social Organization*, chapter 3 (pp. 23-31), New York, 1909.

or community, (2) personal attachment and proximity, and (3) ideological or common cause.[9]

In group (1) the association is based on primary bonds of localism, communalism, and kinship. This intimate association guides status and conduct and thereby limits justice and restrains progress. Its actions have been described as the "antithesis of achievement." Equality is not possible because status is assigned. Because a primary group based on kinship is strong and demands loyalty, it is often considered a restraint on State tyranny. The significance of this threat is seen in authoritarian societies as they attempt to minimize the role of family in acculturation of children. This is occurring in America today. An ancient example was the separation in Sparta of young males from the family unit so that a unified social and military indoctrination and fidelity could be instilled.[10] Dr. Nisbet even noted that primary groups today are "withering away," thereby making the way for totalitarianism.[11] On the other hand, dynastic totalitarianism is common throughout world history, and this often has its leadership and loyalty based on kinship.

In group (2) there is personal attachment and commonality that grows from proximity, but there is no particular orientation toward mutual goals or welfare.

In group (3) there is a common cause and ideology. This group was used to describe activist political and religious groups as they worked to approach their social "ideal." This type of primary group, like group (1), while at times helpful in forwarding a cause, is potentially destructive in its attempts to attain an ideological goal that may be unattainable and because it may introduce schisms that interfere with cohesive solutions for the rest of society.

It is therefore proposed herein that, for primary group (3), "common cause" be considered distinct from "ideology" and placed in a group of its own, *i.e.,* a group (4), and that the common cause be more closely defined as "common council," with collaboration toward a common goal based on self-betterment. Henceforth, the historical group of interest herein is the collaborative group, not one based on emotion, ideology, faith, proximity or kinship.[12]

In summary, group (1) is incompatible with progress, group (2) is neutral, and group (3) is limited to ideology. None of these is helpful in furthering progress, and group (1) is distinctly inhibitory. Focus is now on a new primary group (4), common council based on self-betterment.

---

[9] This pattern of small groups is a modification of those presented in *The Small Group* (New York, 1959, p. 53*ff*), by Dr. Michael S. Olmsted, although it was originally posed by Dr. Edward A. Shils in *Primordial, Personal, Sacred and Civil Ties*, in *Brit. J. Sociol.*, 8:130-145, 1957.

[10] Knottnerus, J. D., and Berry, P. E., *Spartan Society: Structural Ritualization in an Ancient Social System*, in *Humboldt J. Soc. Relations*, 27:1-41, 2002.

[11] Nisbet, R., *The Quest for Community*, 1953.

[12] In *The Natural State of Medical Practice*, volume 1 (pp. 168-175), the ancient Greek koinon (κοινόν) is described as basically an acephalous and voluntary autonomous and democratic group allied by individual self-interest and acting in common council. It was suggested that such a group was formed by a few medical practitioners, and one result was that its shared medical wisdom would be incorporated into the *Hippocratic Corpus*. The koinon would fit perfectly into primary group (4), the common council group.

Importance of common council groups

Collaborative common council groups foster progress, unlike other types of primary groups. Often the common council group has a specific goal, the solving of some particular problem or advancing a particular process, the solution of which would help the members of the group enhance their individual effectiveness in their respective enterprises. Examples might include a group of farmers implementing an irrigation system, a group of medical practitioners forming a local medical association to share clinical information so that each member could be a better doctor, and a corporate research team designing an improved computer chip. The simplest statement explaining the effectiveness of a collaborative group is that two heads are better than one in developing and exploiting an idea.[13] But another benefit of a group lies in its greater number experiences with a particular issue, and this affects the validity of conclusions. There is strengthened statistical significance if an issue is based on nine or ten personal experiences rather than two or three. The conclusion is therefore scientifically more sound.

An important feature of the common council group is its focus on a specific problem(s) of a practical nature by persons with special needs, knowledge or experience with the problem at hand who band together for its solution. Thus, primary group (4), in contrast to the other three primary groups, brings together those with both personal interest and a degree of competence for the project.

A consequence of the collaborative common council is that its efforts may provide desired services that benefit the general population. Solving the issue that is the focus of the group will tend to benefit to society at large. The farmers know that irrigation will benefit them personally, but they also know the reason is that their society will desire the fruits of their labor. The nascent medical practitioners know they will have enhanced remuneration with improved service, because they also know that their society wants improved service. Self-betterment is the personal motivation for their projects, but that is only possible if society at large is keen on it. This inescapable reciprocal and mutually beneficial association between self-interest of a capitalistic free market and the public good is often underappreciated.

Such collaborative groups with the goal of self-betterment would not be permitted in a kinship. But mankind's early break with the kinship occurred because people fled the egalitarianism of the kinship for the personal freedoms associated with early urbanization. The nature of a common council group project and its size can be related to population size, and *The Natural State of Medical Practice* suggests a lower limit of about 10,000 persons in an urban setting is sufficient for establishing a medical "profession" by a small group of practitioners that can be a source of progress.[14]

---

[13] Two heads are better than one" is not a new idea, although leave it to modern scholarship to confirm it as true. See: Wooley, A. W., et al., *Collective Intelligence and Group Performance*, in *Current Directions in Psychological Science*, 24:420-424, 2015. And there is the commonsense interpretation of C. S. Lewis: "Two heads are better than one, not because either is infallible, but because they are unlikely to go wrong in the same direction."

[14] In *The Natural State of Medical Practice* (volume 3, p. 224) and based on evidence, four requirements are proposed:
  1. A collegial network of at least several medical practitioners
  2. Two or three centuries of relative social stability
  3. Prosperity, as evidenced by distant trade and specialized products and services

The pooling of competence in a collaborative group may result in lower costs and quicker service. But its most important consequence is a new or improved product. **And it is the search for a new or improved product that is the basis for scientific discovery and thereby progress.** Tocqueville recognized this process under way in America two hundred years ago. Should the goal of a new or improved product be reached and benefits of discovery or invention become available to the general population of an early society, we would have been privileged to observe the source of progress and an early step toward a true civilization!

At the core of the primary collaborative group, or common council, must be its independence and motivation of self-betterment. Other types of groups with social goals often include within their compass some elements of common council.

Common council and competence

The underlying argument of *The Natural State of Medical Practice*, supported by objective and circumstantial evidence, is that authoritarian political forces delayed human progress for millennia. Discussed in earlier excursus and briefly reviewed here, this occurred several ways:

a. The initiation of progress can be blocked by the controlling policies of the kinship. Its authoritarian nature is described in detail in volume 3, chapter 11 (p. 238*ff*). The kinship prevents progress because its members are assigned their responsibilities and status within the kinship. As a result and despite its fabled egalitarian nature, there is no opportunity or motivation for the innovation and self-betterment that is needed for formation of small autonomous groups necessary for specialization.

b. Discovery and invention by primary collaborative groups once under way, they can be commandeered by political leadership and become the purview of the political hierarchy, which, lacking competency, cannot improve on them. In such a way was rational predynastic Egyptian medicine subsumed by pharaonic priests, never to improve over the next 2500 years.

c. The takeover of a profession or an institution by political leadership also disenfranchises of the bulk of the population because it removes the subsumed profession or institution from choices for the people to improve their status; there is no stimulus to become competent at something. In such a way did Chinese dynastic monarchies bureaucratize their "physicians," thereby diminishing the possibility of a spontaneous reappearance of a profession of rational medicine competitors from the general population.

d. The political leadership, by marginalizing the general population and producing a servile population, blocks the very act of discovering and inventing, checks progress, and thwarts competency. In such a way dynastic kinships of ancient

---

4. A centralized population in the tens of thousands, perhaps as low as 10,000 If the regional environment cannot provide long-term agricultural support for a sedentary population above *ca.* 10,000, the number of independent practitioners will likely be too few from which several could separately agree to collaborate by pooling knowledge for the purpose of improving the service of each member.

China, when they enforced an agricultural culture on a peasant society, removed the capability of self-betterment from ninety percent of its population, a characteristic guaranteeing a society that over three thousand years would be free from progress, getting bigger but not better.

e. Because actions of a centralized political hierarchy are based on politics rather than competency, attempts at logical understanding of adversaries by a dictator represents attempts at reading the mind of other dictators. The incompetence inherent in totalitarian decisions affecting entire societies is proved by their unending wars and destructiveness. A destabilized society is the result, such as contributed to loss of Hippocratic medicine of the Greco-Roman "civilization."

f. The ultimate phase is likely reached when there is no competency in either leadership or the people, with society either becoming subjects of another society and or surviving by conquest. This is a logical prediction, but not an evidence-based conclusion.

Given the social processes that unintentionally prevented progress in ancient times, it is a wonder that progress ever occurred. But occur it did following the Reformation in Europe when increasingly liberal legislation protecting natural rights released the pervasive competence of the unprivileged citizenry.

> Competent: having requisite ability[15]
> Antonym: incompetent

Competency does not require an unusual attribute or unusual intelligence, ability, diligence, strength or cleverness. It requires only a level of ability and motivation considered sufficient to perform a particular task. Many trades, services and professions, through certification, guarantee competency of their members. Competency is distributed throughout the citizenry. In agriculture the farmer is the competent, in transport the trucker is the competent. There is, however, no certification required for political positions, and candidates for political positions cannot be judged competent or incompetent by established standards. It is common to hear a politician being criticized by political opponents as incompetent, but it will be difficult to have that claim objectively proven. A politician may know how to get things done when in office, but the important issue is what it is that which should be done.

With a myriad of competencies, designated "generic competence," distributed throughout the general population and no gauge for competence in higher echelons of government, it seems to have been a sensible conclusion in ancient Athens during its Golden Age (5th C BC) that for a while all positions of civil authority were best selected by lot ("sortition") rather than appointment or democratic election, except for senior military positions.[16] It worked well for that relatively small population. But it is proposed herewith that more important than apolitical leadership and competent politicians is that the generic competency of the entire society be protected. This requires minimizing the effect of centralized governance on its citizens.

Human progress resides in collaboration in common council by the competent. Thus, limiting the opportunity to develop competency or to build on competency, defining

---

[15] Merriam-Webster.com, https://www.merriam-webster.com/dictionary/competent
[16] Herodotus, *The Histories*, Bk. 3, 80.6.

competency in terms of what leadership decides is useful for society, or directing generic competency toward goals of government will be dead ends for progress.

Concentrating incompetence

The necessary functions of government are varied and there can be no one measure of competence for those holding political office. It is no measure of competence to talk glibly, appear likeable, or be ruthless. For government to acquire competence it must seek the advice of those who are competent in performing the myriad activities within a society. But competency distributed among the common people cannot be transposed to centralized government. Furthermore, competent representatives of major activities throughout society may have opposing ideas. What to do? The answer is to do as little as possible and let the competent work things out by themselves. And it axiomatically follows that, with competency in all sorts of things present throughout the general population and with no mechanism for judging competency of those in power, it is best, from the point of view of society, to consider centralized political power as lacking competence, *i.e.*, it is a locus (but not a focus) of incompetence. This is inevitable rather than disparaging. But the point is, why should power be given to a central government characterized by limited competence if it restricts or ignores opinions, or the contest of opinions, of the competent within the broader society?

Central government is necessary for several reasons, but, limited in competence, it should not be entrusted with issues better left to those who are competent. When it infringes on their domain, central government indirectly blocks the people's attempts at innovation and invention, not to mention its civil service and those dependent on government largess, all of whom are automatically limited in their options for improving their status by attempting self-betterment outside of government. Thus, one prong of progress is broken by expanding the limited competence of governance throughout the citizenry and the other prong is broken by commandeering of venues of the people that in a free society normally should invite invention and discovery. The general population is then being guided into a state of incompetency and dependence. Liberty and ingenuity are the losers. The answer, of course, is to leave competence alone and to consider the ideal government one in which, should a person be asked "Who is the President?," there is a long pause.[17]

Note that the limited competence of centralized governance is not meant as an insult to the leaderships of nations. Incompetence is mathematically unavoidable. Most issues of the populace are manageable at local levels. Thus, the fewer the issues that make it to central governance the better, for it means more decisions are made by those who are competent rather than by their political representatives (particularly desirable in medical practice), and central governance can more thoroughly consider those few problems it must necessarily handle and thereby increase its competence in their management.

The considered approach in the preceding paragraph does not, of course, apply to power of the State when it has been assigned to one person. That this medieval, indeed

---

[17] It might be argued that career politicians, rather than term-limited politicians, are an answer to the dearth of centralized competency, for competency should come with experience and deliberative bodies should act as common councils. But governance of a society should not be a playground for self-interests of politicians who can thereby competently proceed to formalize and embed those self-interests into law affecting all of society, although truly deliberative democratic bodies can indeed be considered common councils.

primeval, concept of a supreme leader keeps emerging reflects the power of propaganda and imposed ignorance characteristic of totalitarian societies.

It is, therefore, of greatest concern in the United States that over the past century (1) the power of federal government has vastly increased, thus putting more and more power in the hands of persons whose competence cannot be established and who, for political reasons, often do not assiduously consider the opinion of the truly competent, and (2) the tentacles of government have spread to the point of takeover or control of major segments of our industrial, medical, commercial establishments and blunted the effectiveness of our energy, agriculture, and environmental management. The role of local associations is now minimal. Options for progress are quickly narrowing, compounded by misinformation and overt propaganda via modern technology.

Tocqueville's broad statement on American associations is a statement for the ages. He declares autonomous associations to be the mechanism of progress and the barricade against tyranny. Progress requires competency, not legislation. Authoritarianism is a harbor for the incompetent, and those in government often include many who cannot manage in the world of the competent.

To conclude this section, it is relevant that the issue of competency of centralized governance applies to all governments. Adversarial governments each have the same defects. Thus, problems are actually worse than they seem and more unpredictable whenever two bastions of incompetency come face to face.

Ingenuity and natural law: Linked in freedom

Just as with our conscience and its codified guidance, natural law, we have inherent ingenuity. Like natural law, which protects us from each other, it is human ingenuity that protects us from everything else.

As a general statement, all humans are endowed with equivalent intellectual potential, and from this it can be surmised that the same can be said about ingenuity, although the nature of that ingenuity and the opportunity to express it will vary from person to person.[18] It is an easy assumption that ingenuity is present for a purpose, and that is to serve the individual in whom it resides. Presumably from the very beginning it was meant to ease the path forward for mankind. The sad history of mankind, however, is the history of those who would have that path blocked. *The Natural State of Medical Practice* reveals such a history as it has applied to medicine.

Ingenuity, "the ability to invent things or solve problems in a new way," is a mechanism useful for human survival and benefit. It is a facet of cognitive reasoning and is not learned, although it is applied to things we have learned as we seek to improve or change them. Through reason we understand; in a sense it is passive. Through ingenuity we achieve a goal; it is active. But, as concluded in volume 3 of *The Natural State of Medical Practice* (p. 199*ff*) regarding life expectancy, data do not support the value of ingenuity to our survival as a species. Life expectancy and a superior style of living did not seem any better for the bulk of our ancient ancestors than for other mammalian species

---

[18] "Reason" might be considered interchangeable with "ingenuity," but the former is a frontal lobe function that is a general term that includes intelligence as a measurable quantity used to distinguish among humans, whereas the latter is applied to a specific function (utility). "Ingenuity" rather than "reason" is the focus of this section. Ingenuity can also be equated with "genius" as discussed in the Prologue and p. 205 of *The Natural State of Medical Practice* (vol. 1).

and did not improve over millennia for which there are data. Ingenuity is with us, therefore, for a reason other than just personal survival. Indeed, it seems that its usefulness to survival requires a co-factor to operate, *i.e.*, it is a "potential" benefit that will become manifest when appropriately used, and that benefit can then be made manifest through our society. What is the permissive element?

It is proposed that the permissive element for expression of ingenuity is the collaborative group acting in common council. While an ingenious idea can benefit the individual and those in proximity, it is through the collaborative group of competent persons motivated by self-betterment that an idea can evolve and proliferate to the benefit of both the one and the many. It is through the collaborative common council that the field of medicine has, in the past two centuries been associated with the mean life expectancy of all social classes in many regions around the globe to increase from less than forty to eighty years.

In a sense it is like natural law. It protects our existence as a society just as natural law protects us as individuals. And it is like natural law in that it applies to institutions as well as to individuals. Institutions should not transgress natural law and institutions should not transgress (impede or mismanage) human ingenuity. There will be a price to pay. Authoritarian governance ignores natural law by taking from individuals what they do not want to give, and it ignores human ingenuity when it restricts the options of its citizenry from pursuing self-betterment.

The fact that ingenuity becomes of value to humankind when exploited by a collaborative common council group may be relevant in another way. A malevolent person has his share of ingenuity but can use it to wrong purpose. But if several people recognize or agree to develop an ingenious idea it is less likely to be accidentally or purposely used for ill. Perhaps this is a way of fostering good rather than bad things. Making it necessary for several persons to agree on something may not always make it a better idea, but it may make it safer and help prevent its being used for evil. It is even to be considered that this is one of the principal reasons for the superiority of democratic governance. Not only is democracy a mechanism for exposing the better idea and, by the very fact of its existence, a way of excluding many forms of authoritarian governance; it also may vet an idea as good or evil, presumably by bringing the consciences of many persons into its assessment, *i.e.*, in a free society democracy facilitates the implementation of natural law. Without common council more wild and dangerous ideas might be let loose to proliferate within a society, a common phenomenon in totalitarian states.

Liberty is not just a nice thing to have because it is our birthright or because it allows us to enjoy doing what we want without being harangued. What this discussion brings to the fore is that liberty is essential for our protection and very survival. When our ability to freely associate and collaborate in common council groups on all issues is restricted, we are weakened and our survival as a society is threatened. A society with limitations on responsible freedom is putty in the hands of those leaders who, now in the position of being able to define what is good and evil, have no restrictions as to the use of those definitions to manipulate society.

To conclude, we know that we have natural rights to life, liberty, and pursuit of happiness. But authoritarian governance, whether in a kinship or a nation and even if it does not directly deny life, liberty and pursuit of happiness, can do so indirectly and can thereby prevent human progress and threaten survival.[19] It is one of the many benefits

---

[19] A government that fosters war can lead to great loss of life, thus indirectly denying life to many. A government that appropriates a segment of a national economy indirectly denies liberty to many

following the Reformation that for the first time in human history we have been able to become civilized for an extended period and as individuals to enjoy the security and longevity available in our "Western" civilization.[20] Without the trend to democratic governance and protection of natural rights following the Reformation, the life expectancy for the common man and woman would still be in the mid-thirties. Instead, in the last two centuries billions of lives have been improved because we have the ability to defend ourselves against adverse events of all kinds. Self-betterment is not limited to doing what we want to be "happy." It is the mechanism by which we identify needs and threats and then formulate with others a reasoned solution, one that extends its benefits to society as a whole. But Tocqueville's keen observation on the value to freedom and prosperity of the myriad associations in the United States will be lost to history if expansion of government power and influence continues to build but more paddocks for the common man and woman.

---

who, in common council, would have deliberated and managed issues of that segment on their own, and better. A government that distributes largess (usually with a hitch) to retain power indirectly removes or limits motivation for self-betterment, and the nature of the latter is unique for each individual.

[20] Excursus 16 will pursue further the concept of civilization, the uniqueness of our own, its origin and its name.

EXCURSUS 16

An analysis of our present civilization, often identified as "Western," affirms the importance of the Reformation as its source. The Reformation was preceded by a thousand years without progress in the West, at least in medicine, and therefore was a period classifiable more as a culture than a civilization. But the catalyst of the Reformation exposed the Decalogue as an ethical guide not just for individuals but for governance as well, and it is the latter that has led to Western progress and the Constitution and Bill of Rights of the United States. The Decalogue, transmitted to the ancient Israelites, brought to the fore the primary requirements for a progressive civilization, but demography did not provide the ancient Israelites with the opportunity to formally establish a civilization. This was remedied in the post-Reformation West when Jewish and Christian contributions to civil liberties made it possible to instill progress into our own society (see Excursus 14). Mosaic history thereby became part of our own. It is concluded that there has been only one true mature civilization, the Judeo-Christian civilization. Its global recognition and replication augur well for mankind's future if the Decalogue continues to guide both the individual and the State.

NAMING OUR CIVILIZATION

Introduction

Strictly speaking, who needs a civilization? Why try to fabricate one as if it is, in itself, a good thing? In *The Natural State of Medical Practice* it was proposed, based on evidence, that humans prefer to be free from the harangues of others. Given a safe and fertile environment the natural response is to spread out in individual homesteads or hamlets. Tribal and kinship affiliations are strong in an inhospitable environment, but absent those hazards we prefer to be left alone among our intimates except to celebrate special occasions.

But in difficult environments, as was the usual case in ancient times, only when an acceptable alternative presented itself, such as the commercial settlement with its promise of an easier and more predictable life, did people leave their kinships. It is a logical conclusion, therefore, that early civilizations were not the result of central planning directed toward some wholesome communal end. They were, instead, the natural consequence of people looking to improve their lives by leaving the egalitarian kinship; *i.e.*, civilizations begin with the actualization of human liberty and the opportunity to improve one's life rather than continue in a defined status within the kinship dedicated to maintaining a *status quo* that improves the life of others. Fortunately for human progress, civilizations exist, occasionally.

In *The Natural State of Medical Practice* it was concluded that only six true civilizations can be identified and, of the five ancient ones, four disappeared within a few centuries as they metamorphosed into serial dynastic totalitarian States or were subsumed by other authoritarian political organizations.[1] The sixth is our own, which is in jeopardy.

---

[1] The fifth civilization, the Indus River Valley civilization (flourished 2500-1900 BC), probably declined for geo-climatic reasons, although its intellectual heritage as expressed in the Vedas and ayurveda would subsequently become the basis of Hinduism and Ayurvedic medicine. The other four include the Mesopotamian, Egyptian, Chinese, and Greco-Roman. For present purposes the reason only six civilizations are identified as progressive is because extant rational medical writings

C. S. Lewis would perhaps not find the exposition and characterization of "civilization" presented in *The Natural State of Medical Practice* too far from his own. He pointed out that civilizations are rare, "attained with difficulty and easily lost," and that "the normal state of humanity is barbarism." [2]

As for a definition, Lewis considered civilization "the realization of the human idea." The Isagorial Theory of Human Progress derived from *The Natural State of Medical Practice* urges that some manifestation of progress be included in its definition, with progress being improvement of the human condition as a result of human reason as expressed through collaborative groups. A formal definition of "civilization," as developed from the analysis presented in *The Natural State of Medical Practice*, is:

> "An autonomous urban and rural population sufficiently large to require a regulatory hierarchy to optimize production of a food surplus and trade that contributes to wealth and permits specialization of crafts and vocations capable of progress to the benefit of all citizens."

Consonant with Lewis, "specialization of crafts and vocations" and the progress therefrom, such as is shown in an analysis of medical practice over the ages, are attributes of human reason.

Other definitions of "civilization" abound and, being inordinately subjective, are of little value outside the context described by their authors. But for brevity, civilization has been defined as "being civilized," "a complex rather than simple society," and the "opposite of barbarism and chaos." By these criteria, therefore, a civilization is not barbarous, primitive and static. It is civil, inventive, and progressive, the latter characterized by "gradual betterment" (from Merriam-Webster, the noun "progress," definition 3). Without the ability to progress it is little more than a club. In that it is the consequence of human reason in a dangerous world, civilization is desirable. Whether or not it is necessary is indeterminate. To assist in understanding of this excursus, it is helpful to have read about primary and other "civilizations" in Excursus 14.

Civilizations of today

Current civilizations, according to Dr. Arnold Toynbee in mid-20th century, include Western Christian, Orthodox-Russian, Orthodox-Byzantine, Islamic, Hindu, Chinese and Far Eastern.[3] More recently there seems to be some hesitation in listing modern civilizations. In part this is because what is called "Western" civilization has left its mark globally with the proliferation of technology and the spread of Christianity, blurring the uniqueness of global cultures over the last two centuries. Nevertheless, this has not restrained some from anticipating characteristics of civilizations yet to be. Nikolai Kardashev proposed a scaling of civilizations based on technology as gauged by energy

---

can be traced to their earliest stages, thus allowing some objective assessment of civilizational progress. That as yet unidentified true civilizations could have originated elsewhere and at other times is acknowledged.

[2] C. S. Lewis, *Our English Syllabus*, in *Rehabilitations and Other Essays*, London, 1939, pp. 82-83.

[3] This list is identified by Dr. Toynbee in his 1934 volume 1 Introduction of his famous 12-volume *A Study of History*.

production.[4] Others anticipate a single global civilization, and some even suggest it is already upon us. The role of artificial intelligence is debated.

Dr. Samuel Huntington (1927-2008) identified eight contemporary civilizations. While pointing out their differing ideologies and the historically recent opportunity to further advance themselves apart from the West and thereby potentiating a "clash of

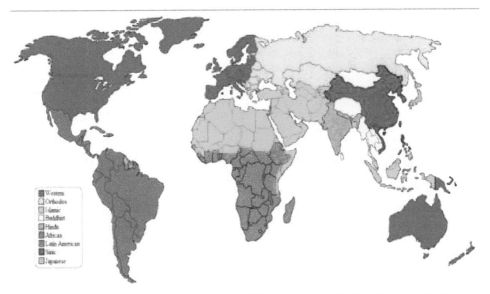

Figure: Contemporary civilizations, from Samuel Huntington (1996), *The Clash of Civilizations and the Remaking of World Order.*

civilizations," they can also be defined by geography.[5] If there are any smaller civilizations, they are subsumed by those that dominate regional geography. The notable feature of Huntington's list of civilizations is the association of most with a dominant culture identified with religion: Western Christian, Orthodox Christian, Hinduism, Buddhism, and Islam, with South and Latin America, Japan, and southern Africa separately considered (this is similar to Toynbee's earlier list mentioned in the preceding paragraph). It is interesting today to note his prediction in 1996 of fault-lines between civilizations as locations for future conflict, for among the modern countries he would locate on fault-lines are Israel, Ukraine, Nigeria, Sudan, Afghanistan, Chechnya and Pakistan, all locations presently threatened or contested by arms.

Judaism, which Dr. Toynbee considered a fossilized culture, Dr. Huntington generally avoided. This may have been unfair, as the following will argue.

---

[4] See: Balega, Y. Y., et al., *In Memory of Nikolai Semenovich Kardashev*, in *Physics-Uspekhi*, 63:622-624.
[5] Samuel P. Huntington, *The Clash of Civilization and the Remaking of World Order*, New York, 1996. The Figure of the civilizations is copied from that book.

The uniqueness of our civilization and its origin

Excursus 14 explored how "civilization" is to be defined. After requiring that the term "progress" be included in the definition, it settled on the disquieting conclusion that there is only one true civilization that has achieved a degree of maturity, our own. It is only in the West that progress took hold, producing the means for a more secure, healthful and longer life expectancy that has spread globally to help billions of people.

In *The Natural State of Medical Practice* (volume 1, p. 439*ff*), modern medical progress was shown to originate in the post-Reformation West, *i.e.*, since the 16th C. It was not a continuation of Hippocratic medicine from ancient Greece or any other ancient source because the intervening thousand years of Dark Age and Medieval medicine had, in effect, no professional practitioners worthy of the name. That particular millennium of European history does not seem to represent any civilization in that it was feudal, static, and unable to progress. Nevertheless, the underlying benevolence of its unifying common religion suggests its designation as a Christian *culture*.

But once underway in the 18th C, modern medical practice has justifiably been referred to as Western medicine. It seems logical, therefore, to consider it a manifestation of a Western civilization. And, as cultural and institutional components of the Dark Ages and Medieval period merged into our contemporary civilization, it seems reasonable to combine the Western and Christian aspects into a single civilization that can be dated from the early centuries of the 1st millennium AD, as Drs. Toynbee and Huntington proposed. It is to be noted, however, that the Dark Ages and Medieval period did not contain the seeds of progress. As will be explained below, the only reason they can justifiably be retained as part of a Christian civilization is that they serve as a conduit of Christian history and culture that connects the Torah with the present.

It was also proposed in *The Natural State of Medical Practice* that a common distinguishing feature associated with the other five nascent, or "primary," civilizations as well as our own was a level of civil liberty and prosperity of sufficient duration that permitted specialization, thus enabling medical progress to appear. The critical role of civil liberty raises a question: how did that freedom arise? For the five ancient early civilizations the explanation is obvious: the absence of an authoritarian political hierarchy during the settlement hierarchy phase of early urbanization. Thus left alone, humans will invent, discover, and, if demographics suffice, progress.

This, however, is not an adequate explanation for our own civilization, for it evolved in a large European region divided among thousands of feudal dominions and culturally contained by the Vatican's dominant leadership of a super-kinship, the Roman Catholic Church. Thus, political authoritarianism and kinship were combined in resisting any claim to civil liberty. From where and how did such freedom arise that led to the flowering of progress in medicine that began in the 18th C?

The Natural State of Medical Practice concluded the critical event to be the 16th C Protestant Reformation that for convenience can be dated to 1517 and the internal revolution in the Church instigated by Martin Luther. The explanation was felt not to lie to any great extent in the evolving Protestant work ethic that supposedly fostered capitalism. It rather was integration of the Decalogue of the Torah into the political sphere that reformed political hierarchies to accommodate increasingly democratic governance and recognition of natural rights.

This transposition was not sudden. Human history is filled with anecdotal evidence of attempts at freedom of conscience and liberty of the individual. Furthermore, the issue is complex. But there is an evolutionary thread that ties the two together, and that is adherence to *natural law*. Both Luther (1483-1546) and Calvin (1509-1564) considered natural law and the Decalogue (*ca.* 1300 BC) to be equivalents, thus providing a common three-thousand-year-old referent for the following sections.[6]

The Decalogue in prehistory and history, a summary

Modern explications and criticisms of the Decalogue, while thought-provoking and varied, are more complex than necessary for this excursus. This is in part because of the iconic status it has acquired in the centuries following its appearance in *Exodus* 20, which some estimate at 1300 BC; *i.e.,* its importance rests not only on what it says, but also what it has come to mean. A recent summary by Dr. Leon R. Kass concerning the origin, contemporary and iconic significance of the Decalogue includes a division between those Commandments that specify the relation of people to God, the ritual Commandments, and those that guide the relation of members of a society to one another, the ethical Commandments, the latter being more directly relevant here.[7]

The Decalogue is considered a moral guide, and its message is restated in natural law. And natural law is there to protect our natural rights. They include our rights to life, to property, and to liberty. The latter comprises no transgression of family, reputation or, by implication, way of life. The Decalogue did not identify "liberty" or "civil liberty" as a natural right. To explicitly specify individual liberty as a natural right would have been incomprehensible to the ancient world and instantly ridiculed and forgotten. To live outside the kinship or totalitarian unit was irrational. Thus, the concept of individual civil liberty seems justifiably unspecified in the Decalogue, and that particular interpretation would not make itself understood by mankind until after the Reformation. In the interim, the Decalogue was considered solely as a religious guide for the individual in society, Commandments from God that good people should obey. Civil allegiance, a separate issue, was to one's leader, tribe, or clan, and to not acknowledge some such association

---

[6] See Calvin, *In Rom*, ad 2.14-15, 46. "He indeed shows that ignorance is in vain pretended as an excuse by the Gentiles, since they prove by their own deeds that they have some rule of righteousness: for there is no nation so lost to every thing human, that it does not keep within the limits of some laws. Since then all nations, of themselves and without a monitor, are disposed to make laws for themselves, it is beyond all question evident that they have some notions of justice and rectitude, which the Greeks call preconceptions προληψεις, and which are implanted by nature in the hearts of men. They have then a law, though they are without law: for though they have not a written law, they are yet by no means wholly destitute of the knowledge of what is right and just; as they could not otherwise distinguish between vice and virtue; the first of which they restrain by punishment, and the latter they commend, and manifest their approbation of it by honoring it with rewards. He sets nature in opposition to a written law, meaning that the Gentiles had the natural light of righteousness, which supplied the place of that law by which the Jews were instructed, so that they were a law to themselves." Translation by vicar John Owen (1788-1868) of Calvin's text (here partially supplied in Latin because of its great importance to subsequent events):
"Nulla enim gens vnquam sic ab humanitate abhorruit vt non se intra leges aliquas contineret. Quum igitur sponte ac sine monitore, gentes omnes ad leges sibi ferendas inclinatae sunt, constat absque dubio quasdam iustitiae ac rectitudinis conceptiones quas Graeci prolhyei~ vocant hominum animis esse naturaliter ingenitas. Habent ergo legem sine Lege."
[7] Dr. Leon R. Kass, *The Ten Commandments: Why the Decalogue Matters*, in *Mosaic Magazine*, June 3, 2013

would have been unthinkable.[8] To not "leave unto Caesar what is Caesar's" would have been a wild idea to contemporaries. This was convenient for political authorities, who would claim that allegiance and proceed with "positive" (man-made) laws they deemed appropriate for regulating society rather than trying to make do with just the Ten Commandments. The Decalogue was viewed as a one-way street; common people were to obey, but governance had no such obligation.

But the Decalogue's protection of individual rights transcended the kinship or other social agency. Its full implementation was directed at *both* the individual and the society. Yes, a person is to obey the Commandments, but everyone else is to do the same, and therefore this means individual rights are protected from transgression by society as a whole, including its leadership. Not only is it a guide for all people; none benefit inordinately from its implementation. It favors everyone and no one more than another, and it clearly is not a statement issued by a temporal ruler, for there is no benefit via power or wealth that one or a few person(s) can claim or accrue if that ruler also follows those Commandments. This contrasts with the law codes of Hammurabi and Ur-Nammu, and is an argument for its Divine nature.

It is therefore somewhat of a surprise that the message of the Decalogue has only recently been politically codified, specifically on March 4th, 1789. It is also a condemnation of all rulers prior to the *Constitution of the United States* and its *Bill of Rights* for abusing their privileges as leaders by not implementing it, or at least accommodating it. Had they done so, humanity would have bettered its health, security and longevity much earlier.[9] While we are now enjoying the remarkable benefits of our natural rights, it is important to remember that their overwhelming importance to us as individuals resides in the individual's protection from society; *i.e.*, in a civic setting the Commandments are, in effect, the obligations of others so that our own natural rights are protected.

The Decalogue can now be viewed as a fulfillment of the religious Covenant between God and the Israelites but on a broader scale. A religious interpretation might suggest that if we are true to the Commandments, God will see that we prosper. What was missing prior to the Reformation was recognition of the importance of governance of society as a whole in obeying the Decalogue. Would that it had been obvious.

---

[8] Dr. Ralph Lutz, in his article *The History of the Concept of Freedom* in *Bull. of the Amer. Assoc. of Univ. Prof.*, 36:18-32, 1950, dates the concept of civil liberties with the democracies of ancient Greece. That may not be accurate. The democracies in ancient Greece were oriented toward survival of the city-state rather than individual freedom, with voting and other aspects of Greek democracy thereby enlisted as motivating factors to increase personal stake in city-state protection. "As a [Greek] citizen decided peace and war, as a private individual, he was constrained, watched and repressed in all his movements; as a member of the collective body, he interrogated, dismissed, condemned, beggared, exiled, or sentenced to death his magistrates and superiors; as a subject of the collective body he could be deprived of his status, stripped of his privileges, banished, put to death, by the discretionary will of the whole to which he belonged." Benjamin Constant (1767-1830), *The Liberty of the Ancients Compared to That of the Moderns* [De la Liberte des Anciene Comparee a Celle des Modernes], a speech given in Paris, 1819. Constant was of Huguenot descent and received his education in part from the University of Edinburgh. This excursus therefore places the concept of civil liberties as post-Reformation.

[9] No society is perfect, even one with constitutional protections of natural rights, and it took a terrible civil war to ensure that all citizens of the United States had that legal protection, although issues of implementation have, and probably always will, bedevil interpretation of the Constitution.

In addition to the Decalogue's regulations for society, Judaism from its earliest days stressed the equality of all people before God; we were made in the image of God and we are descended from God's creations, the first man and woman. This fostered a classless society and an egalitarian impulse in Judaism that has existed ever since. This same impulse helped initiate the Reformation when Martin Luther profoundly announced that every member of the Church was equal to Church leaders in the eyes of God.

In conclusion, following the Reformation there were two remarkable social developments over the next two centuries: (1) increasing recognition of natural rights for all people, and (2) extension of natural law to the civil sphere. Thus, secular leaders were to be limited in their privileges and the common citizenry were not to have their natural rights transgressed. Furthermore, not often mentioned but most important for progress, those civil liberties and protections extended to *everyone*. The great mass of humanity was encompassed in the event, not just the leaders, kings, chiefs, King John's nobles and gentry. With hierarchical political power on a grand scale now being restrained for the first time in the history of the world, the ingenuity of humanity was released *en mass* in the West, and progress ensued. In part because of its association with Judaism and Christianity and in part because it has become so prominent in Western political thought, the ethical Decalogue has, with global expansion of modern progress emanating from the West, permanently ensconced itself as the iconic declaration of human freedom for all time.[10]

---

[10] Uncertain is the status of Islam in this iconization of the Decalogue. Moses and the Commandments are duly acknowledged, praised and implemented by the Quran, for specific statements in the Quran consistent with the Decalogue have been identified. If the Decalogue can be credited as the permissive agent for human progress, why should not Islam be included in our civilization's name? And Islam would seem to have had a head start in that in its early centuries prominent cities and scholars emerged at a time when Europe was feudal, static and unable to progress. On the other hand, elements of the Quran clearly inconsistent with the Decalogue have been noted (see for example *Islam and the Decalogue* by Prof. Howard Kainz, published in *The Catholic Thing* (July 23, 2016). The essential difference seems to be Islamic resistance to extending the social protections inherent in the Decalogue to "nonbelievers."

There are historical similarities between the Roman Catholic Church and Islam. Neither has been friendly to the other, particularly evident in the Christian Crusades sanctioned by the Pope and the westward extensions of the Ottoman Empire that conquered Constantinople and ended the Byzantine Empire. Power emanated from the top: the Pope (and his interactions with the Holy Roman Emperor) in the former, the Sultan in the latter. Dependent regions were, in both, subjects of a "super-kinship" based on religion, with all the baggage that a kinship carries that functions to prevent progress. Islam split into various factions over the centuries, and the Church also had unruly factions.

Islam was reaching its zenith early in the 16th C under Suleiman the Magnificent, whereas at about the same time the Roman Catholic Church experienced a dramatic schism, the Reformation. Perhaps a justification for not including Islam as a component of our Western civilization can be traced to the reasons for the Reformation, for this resulted in separation of large populations, especially northern Europe, from the "believers" in the Roman Catholic Church. The former were considered heretics rather than nonbelievers, but over the next three centuries it was northern and western Europe that would carry the Reformation forward, advance civil liberties and natural rights, and be the spearhead for progress of our Western civilization.

Fractures occurred in the Islamic world as well. But at the time of the Reformation the Ottoman Empire was reaching its greatest extent and influence, its leadership and economy in the hands of the Osman dynasty, Sufism its State creed, and its goal to extend its borders and advance Islam. There was no popular uprising against the power of that Empire. Thus, the earliest major

The primacy of the Decalogue

Dr. John Witte, Jr., has provided an enlightening scholarly narrative describing the sequential changes in the social and political implications of the Reformation.[11] Prodded by violent events in Europe, the maturation of political thought during its first century affected the political implications of the Decalogue and the political prominence of Calvinists in the Old World and the New. From this political thinking changes in governance came ever closer to an equivalence between church leadership and its laity and government leadership and its people. Leaders in both instances were being viewed as no more important than the people they led, government should follow the same rules as the individual, replaceable if they did not, and behind the curtain and offering guidance for all were the Commandments.

Calvinists from the beginning recognized the importance of separation of church and state and the responsibility for correcting unjust positive laws and "overbearing tyranny." Although the great importance in maintaining public order was stressed, an individual's rights to property and other aspects of daily life were accepted, based on Calvin's interpretation of biblical statements contemporary with Roman law. It was also considered that natural law applied to everyone, believers and non-believers, and provided "civil norms" relevant to governance. Within the church, freedom to assemble, debate and elect was not to be restricted. Dr. Witte concludes, "Calvin described natural law as a set of moral commandments, written on the heart, repeated in the Scripture, and summarized in the Decalogue."[12]

The Decalogue's political importance was specifically stated by Christopher Goodman in 1558:

> Yf you therfore be Gods subjects and people, and he your Lorde God and
> louing Father, who is aboue all powers ad Princes, ad hath made no Lawes,
> but such as are for your preseruuation, and singuler comforte: then without
> all controuersie there maye be nothinge lawfull for you by anie commandment
> of man, whiche your Lorde god in anie case forbiddeth: and nothinge vnlawfull

---

attempt at democratizing Islamic regions, which was short-lived, would not appear until late in the 19th C.

It is proposed, therefore, that the reason why modern progress is attributable to the West and Judeo-Christianity but not Islam stems from the Reformation, and a prominent feature of the Reformation was the new interest in the Decalogue which the State was also to obey. Elements of the Decalogue can be found in the Quran, but they are not an inclusive list, instead being implied in scattered statements. Indeed, the specific scriptural citations in the Torah are considered by Islam to be outdated. It appears, therefore, that it is the original Commandments, subjected to intense scrutiny by Judeo-Christian scholars, that can be considered the spark and the fuel for Western progress, whereas Shariah law, while religious in nature and affirming all persons are equal, is extensive and complex, and in its social obligations (*mu aralat*) is oriented to economic/commercial activities and eye-for-an-eye and other aspects of criminal law and punishment. The Decalogue in effect says "Do not do ...," whereas Shariah law says "If you do this ..., then ... ."

[11] Much of the following is based on a foundational chapter by Dr. John Witte, Jr., entitled *Calvinist Contributions to Freedom in Early Modern Europe*, in *Christianity and Freedom*, volume 1, *Historical Perspectives*, Cambridge (UK), 2016, pp. 210-234.

[12] This is extensively discussed in a book also by Dr. John Witte, Jr., *The Reformation of Rights*, 2007, pp. 156-169. He stresses the point that Calvin himself considered the conscience, natural law and the Decalogue to be equivalents.

or forbidden to you whiche he commandeth, whither it appartayne to the firste Table or the Seconde [*i.e.*, the ritual or the ethical Commandments].

From this it is clear that, as Dr. Witte comments, "... a person has the inalienable right to life, to property, to marital integrity, and to reputation and fair process. A person has the inalienable right to be free from having his family household, and possessions coveted by others."

Then followed Theodore Beza (1519-1605) whose writings formalized the rights and responsibilities of the people in the face of tyrannical government. An example of this thinking was the publication *Vindiciae Contra Tyrannos* (1579), from which the name of our website, **contratyrannos.com**, is derived. Thomas Helwys (1575-1616) died in prison for declaring the absolute separation of church and State.[13]

Dr. Witte then describes what might be considered the mature political version of the intellectual process traceable to the Decalogue by reviewing the writings of the eminent jurist, Johannes Althusius (1557-1638). In addition to stating that "The natural law imparts to all men a freedom of the soul or mind," Althusius construed the ethical Laws of the Decalogue to comprise "a full system of public, private, penal and procedural rights" inherent in the positive laws of government. As Dr. Witte grandly concludes, "By the time he was finished, he had defined and defended almost every one of the rights that would appear in the American federal and state constitutions a century and a half later."

This linkage between the Decalogue and the consequences of the Reformation strongly binds the Hebrews of the Old Testament to the Christians of the New Testament. It also binds everyone else to this pairing, for, of utmost significance, the concept of natural law is not limited to the Judeo-Christian religion. The concept is commonl accepted by believers and nonbelievers alike, although the source of natural law is debated. Excursus 6 briefly describes the consensus about the universal presence and applicability of natural law. The only distinction between Judeo-Christian and other formulations of natural law is that the former has now been codified and legislatively implemented to varying degrees in the West whereas elsewhere positive laws have restricted its import.

The reason for the retention and prominence of the Decalogue in the West is attributed by some to its original covenantal nature. This entailed its observance by both parties (*i.e.*, God and the ancient Israelites), whereas the expression of natural law elsewhere was more subtle and readily superseded or camouflaged when convenient by authoritarian positive laws. In the Torah a direct interaction of man with God is palpably obvious and it has purposely remained so for millennia. For present purposes, the Message as given to the ancient Israelites in the Decalogue is without question historically tied to the Reformation and modern Western progress.

Judeo-Christian unification

From the preceding, Israel can be considered part of Huntington's Western Christian civilization even though it is geographically encompassed by Islam in Huntington's global physical partitioning of civilizations (see Figure). But there are those who would assign Judaism to a civilization unto itself spanning 4,000 years and

---

[13] Helwys, Thomas, *A Short Declaration of the Mistery of Iniquity*, 1612.

manifested by a tenacious and robust religious structure and an intercommunicative global diaspora existing within its original religious tenets. Yet the Jewish contribution to modern progress when working in non-Jewish environments in the West has been done hand-in-glove with the latter and the resulting progress contributes to everyone's benefit. Thus, the two come together fairly well in the concept of a Jewish and Christian alliance. This alliance has done what the ancient Jewish people alone were unable to do.

This combination would reset the beginning of our "Western" civilization, for Western Christian civilization is traceable only to the time of Christ or a few centuries later. But with the inclusion of the history of the ancient Hebrews the date of origin of our civilization could now be placed, albeit controversially, to about 1300 BC. Is this a reasonable interpretation of history?

Jewish history begins with a nomadic people and tribal activities regulated by local *edahs*, or councils, and that tendency toward a classless popular governance has persisted ever since. An analysis of its antiauthoritarian roots by Rabbi Robert Gordis is presented in Excursus 8. But an early sedentary and prosperous agricultural existence that might have fostered a nascent civilization with commerce, prosperity, and specialization of beneficial services such as medicine did not develop. An early city of prominence to ancient Hebrews was Shiloh, but it was already the site of an earlier walled Canaan city when the Israelites arrived, and it functioned thereafter as a religious center rather than a commercial one. Thus, neither the early history nor subsequent captivities and dispersions lent themselves demographically to initiation of a primary civilization characterized by progress as proposed and described in *The Natural State of Medical Practice*, volume 3.[14] Without a homeland that could support a sizeable and commercially-based permanent society, Judaism remained dispersed, and captivities, wars and cultural distinctions would prevent merging with another civilization for more than a thousand years.

Scholarship regarding the Decalogue is extensive and ongoing, but for present purposes reference is specifically to the biblical narrative of *Exodus* 20. The uniqueness of the Decalogue has been questioned. Dr. Andrew Wilson has published extensively on the similarities in ideas, including the Decalogue, as expressed in sacred texts of various world religions.[15] It has also been proposed that the similarities between the laws of Moses and those of Hammurabi are such to suggest the former were derived from the latter. Arguments for and against this position have been based on the wording of some of the laws and on the difference in legal context. Differences include: the Hammurabi code is a list of criminal and civil laws whereas Mosaic laws are ethical and religious/ritual in nature, despite similarity of some specific items; the laws of Hammurabi specify punishment, whereas Mosaic laws do not; Mosaic laws are considered apodictic (definitively handed down) and the Hammurabi code is casuistic (based on precedent). Excursus 6 discusses natural law and its expression in many ancient and contemporary societies. It is argued that natural law is an inherent component of the human conscience, and its message is the same as the Decalogue. As mentioned above, this was Calvin's interpretation, and the prominent anthropologist, Dr. Margaret Mead, noted its nearly

---

[14] The matter of the Ten Lost Tribes is unsettled as is their whereabouts, and they are not included in the present considerations.

[15] Dr. Andrew Wilson, *World Scripture: A Comparative Anthology of Sacred Texts*, New York, 1991.

universal presence in contemporary primitive societies.[16] As people of all times and places seem to share this attribute, similarities in its expression in laws, religions and sacred texts of various sorts around the world should come as no surprise.

But it was the Covenant with the Israelites that guaranteed the historical survival of the formal tenets of the Decalogue for future generations. Some might say this happened for a reason: early humankind did not obey its multitude of consciences, in each of which lay inherent knowledge of good and bad, and as a consequence God selected the ancient Israelites for a Covenant with more explicit instructions on the content of natural law, what we call the Decalogue, to oversee that its message was made clear to all mankind. Being insufficiently effective, for whatever reason, in spreading that message, God's Covenant with the Israelites was reinforced by the introduction of Christianity to expand it globally. That unification, in fact, is what has been occurring, regardless of what one might consider its origin.

Our civilization's name

Although the Decalogue and its Hebraic origin remained a popular theme subsequent to the Reformation, it was not Luther who would make room for Jewish inclusion in Western society. It was the demography of an awakening 16th C Europe in which the significance of the individual before God, eloquently defended by Luther, became a guide and justification for civil liberties. Attempts at promoting civil liberties had been unsuccessfully percolating in Europe for centuries.[17] But with the Reformation this pairing of individualism and civil liberty now matched the ethos of Jewish populations ensconced throughout Europe. Despite the many centuries of prejudice, fear, envy and malice that periodically had wreaked havoc on their communities, by the 18th C Jewish contributions to society in commerce, art, and science were recognized, appreciated and rewarded. This was not done by edict and it was not done by some sudden change of heart. It represented instead the opening of European society to the significance of individual rights and natural law that made it easier to overlook cultural differences, making them objects of interest and merit rather than emblems of peculiarity and division. The Jewish ethos and Protestant ethos seemed so different yet were so similar because of the Decalogue that previous "tribal" distinctions lost their perceived importance as their true importance became manifest. England was especially the recipient of this foremost but unanticipated consequence of the Reformation, although it took two centuries to make its mark. It was, therefore, in post-Reformation Europe that Western civilization belatedly made room for an embryonic Jewish civilization that was full of potential but for more than three millennia was lacking in opportunity.

---

[16] Margaret Mead, *Some Anthropological Considerations Concerning Natural Law*, in *Natural Law Forum*, 1961, paper 59, pp. 51-64; http://scholarship.law.nd.edu/nd_naturallaw_forum/59. Also see: James Q. Wilson, *The Moral Sense*, New York, 1993. Dr. Wilson does not equate the moral sense and natural law in his book, but he elsewhere has stated he hoped they were the same (see Acton Institute in *Religion and Liberty*, vol. 9, No. 4, *The Free Society Requires a Moral Sense, Social Capital*). And C. S. Lewis also considered a moral sense to be found in all societies, even primitive ones.

[17] The Magna Carta of 1215 was an early manifestation, one that was annulled within weeks by Pope Innocent III, only later to reemerge somewhat changed.

In addition to political and economic integration, combining Western Christianity with Judaism under the cognomen of a civilization is supported by religious heritage, which under Dr. Huntington's schematic is the principle "cultural" distinction for his eight civilizations.[18] As a result, "civilization," properly defined as having a directional component based on progress, now can include the equivalent Judaic and Western contributions to progress and can claim recognition for the global benefits proceeding therefrom.

The present-day concept of the "West" is so vast, its culture(s) so varied, and its inclusiveness so subjective that as a term it is meaningless to refer to a Western civilization.[19] An alternative designation is needed. When most people use the phrase "Christian" civilization they mean Judeo-Christian. It is therefore not only appropriate but convenient to apply the term "Judeo-Western Christian," or perhaps "Judeo-Western" or, my preference, "Judeo-Christian," to our own civilization, to consider it as the only mature true civilization that has ever existed, and to date its first appearance to the age of the Ten Commandments, almost four thousand years ago.

It remains to be seen if the Judeo-Christian civilization will expand to a single global civilization. The resistance to this intrusion into other cultures will probably be impossible to overcome, and understandably so in the foreseeable future. But the possibility should be considered within a century or so because it is clear that modern benefits of progress to every human being is solely the result of adherence, however tardy, halting, and unintentional as it has been, to the Decalogue, whether in its apodictic form or as natural law, the Golden Rule, or our conscience. It is to the Decalogue of Judeo-Christian religion that we can attribute the civil liberties that have lifted the unprivileged citizenry out of what seemed destined to remain eternal serfdom. It is only because of the Decalogue that power of the political hierarchy has been diminished and the ingenuity of humanity released. Natural law itself was insufficient to do the trick. Unless new information reveals itself and based primarily on the pre-history and history of medical practice, Western progress in health, security and longevity justifies the naming of our civilization the *Judeo-Christian Civilization*. With the proof now in hand the course forward seems obvious.

---

[18] The importance of increased religious tolerance in the interweaving of cultures is discussed by Dr. Mark Koyama in *Persecution and Toleration: The Long Road to Religious Freedom*, Cambridge, 2019. He concluded the decreased status of the Roman Catholic Church, the increased cost and effort at ensuring religious conformity, and the unnecessary nature of ancillary religious services and identity to the citizenry at large combined to favor religious tolerance that flourished in the 18th C.

[19] See Figure on p. 167.

EXCURSUS 17

In an effort to unite the history of medical practice with events and portents of the present day, the appearance and disappearance of rational medicine in ancient civilizations is again reviewed. Focus is on the practitioner over the ages, how medical progress emerged solely from the clinical efforts of the practitioner, and how interference in the practitioner's domain profoundly inhibited medical progress. The mechanisms of that interference are summarized and then shown to be similar to recent events in American medicine. It is concluded that medicine is increasingly under the control of an authoritarian political class, and that intrusion into the physician-patient relation will turn our profession into a trade and restrict clinical progress. Government, *per se*, has never contributed to human progress, but in America constitutional safeguards have protected our natural rights by limiting the role of government. This is being dangerously undermined.

PHYSICIAN OR PHARAOH'S PRIEST; OR ARE WE DOCTORS OR MOUTHPIECES [1]

Introduction

In this disheartening chronicle of medical practice over the ages and its message for today's medicine, the intent is not to predict a return to the tragic history of human society that preceded the rise of Western democracies and modern medicine. We can hope that democracy, individual liberty, and the fact and the concept of progress have so taken hold around the world that, even if we continue to lose or willfully relinquish our freedoms to government, sparks of freedom elsewhere will remain to rekindle the flame of human progress and ultimately remove authoritarian threats forever. It must not be forgotten, however, that, in the century just past, great hope, yearnings and sacrifices for freedom and progress in its early years could quickly turn to utter tragedy. The Russian revolution replaced but one totalitarian with another, Stalin and his communism, and predictably by 1980, despite a century of magnificent medical progress in the contemporary West, Russian medicine was considered the worst in the world.[2] Similarly, the new Chinese republic, during which Dr. Sun Yat-sen attempted a transformation to Western medicine, was replaced by a communist government so that, for economic reasons, by 1970 the Cultural Revolution saw a complete rescinding of Western medicine and a return to purely traditional Chinese medicine as practiced by laymen, the "barefoot doctors." The unwritten tragedies of the hundreds of millions of common men, women and children without the advantages of Western medicine over much of the 20th century in two of the three largest countries in the world would dwarf the unspeakable tragedies of their wars. The world of the authoritarian can turn on a dime. But now to return to the problem at hand.

---

[1] Facts and arguments supporting many statements and conclusions in this excursus can be found in *The Natural State of Medical Practice* published by Liberty Hill Press, Maitland FL, 2019, in three volumes, especially volume 1 and 3.
[2] Consult the *Foundation for Economic Education* and its newsletter of May 2004, for an article by Anna Ebeling, *The Government Dream and the Soviet Reality*.

Many difficult issues beset modern medical practice. It shouldn't be this way. Since mankind's earliest societies it is fundamentally the simplest of arrangements. There are only two people involved, the medical practitioner, hereafter the "physician," and the patient. As they attempt to resolve medical problems, the interaction is highly personal and private, relying on honesty and trust by the participants, the "natural state" of medical practice; no outside interference. The patient's problem is clarified and analyzed by what a former colleague of mine called "a compassionate medical scholar." In turn, the physician's obligation is solely to the patient. The essence of this simple interaction remains unchanged over thousands of years.

But medical practice is changing and changing greatly. Something is imposing itself between the compassionate medical scholar and the patient. What is the context within which clinical practice now finds itself?

The federal government of the United States lists thirty-one "public health" agencies doing its bidding and pays $1.5 trillion (43%) of total U. S. medical costs ($3.5 trillion as of 2019), pharmaceutical companies sell drugs at $500 billion and spend $90 billion on research and development, American hospitals received $1.2 trillion for hospital services (2020), medical devices and instruments amount to about $200 billion, and private health coverage was $1.1 trillion (2020). To this can be added liability, medical schools, and other medically related costs.

Popular attention is typically directed to all these massive activities and agencies, but it is the physician-patient relation that is the reason for their very existence. Intrusive forces that target the daily work of the clinician are too diffuse to be quantified, and it is no wonder that physicians are so often caught up in administrative and legal process. Indeed, it is to the credit of physicians that their work, both in its implementation and in its public image, still maintains strong ties with the Hippocratic Oath. And the reasons for this so far are public expectation of the profession's adherence to the Oath and the successful defensive posture by many in medicine against powerful forces that try to infringe on our profession and drive it beyond its justifiable borders.

The medical profession also knows that the responsibility that goes with managing trillions of dollars, giant industries, political machines and national meetings is minor when compared to the responsibility of working with a sick patient. With the former, salary and working hours are good and predictable. Moreover, responsibility for most decisions is conveniently and diffusely distributed among many persons, and personal blame for bad results can therefore be disclaimed or off-loaded onto others, especially opponents. This of course is one of the great appeals of committees; dispersion of responsibility. But in the physician's office responsibility is solely the prerogative of the physician, and it has truly been said that "You can't practice medicine by committee." There is justification for a degree of contempt for external compulsion intruding on our profession. Medical progress is not promoted by meddling with the physician-patient relation; that is where medical progress indisputably begins. Most physicians know this, but it is difficult if faced with legislative actions by a government backed by force.

It must be made clear at the outset that the history and physical examination in the physician's office is the basis for everything in medicine: not only the clinical diagnosis, prognosis, and agreement on therapy, but also outside the office: the tools of medicine for diagnosis, the therapies of medicine, the indications for their use, the specialized services of other healthcare providers, the research for new preventives and treatments, the pharmaceutical companies, the medical device companies, organizational necessities such as hospitals, insurance, public health, ambulance services, physician training, State Boards to set standards of practice, and on and on. Were it not for the interaction of the physician and patient in the physician's office, none of these agencies or activities would have a reason to exist. There is no more *sanctum sanctorum* of secular interfaces in human society than the physician's office.

But it is *sanctus* no more. Government-sponsored organizations now have extensive control over the practice of medicine. Regulations and committees have opened the physician's office and patient interaction to public view despite signs and instructions posted everywhere claiming the opposite. The only activity that for the most part benefits from, but manages to keep out of the way of, the physician's business is capitalistic enterprise. There can be seemingly relentless enticements, and clinical trials can affect the care of some patients (although only with their concurrence after evaluation of risk/benefit), but it is capitalism and its intrinsic goal of personal betterment that takes its cue from findings of medical practitioners as to what is needed. At that point the magic of capitalism develops, improves, and distributes the needed [thing] even on a global scale to the benefit of mankind. All else is obstacle, some necessary, many not.

In the criticisms that will emanate from this excursus, I must acknowledge that I have limited personal experience with government regulation of medical practice. Before my retirement in 2002 I was on the staff of Harlem Hospital in New York City, and it was to the credit of that hospital that clinical decisions were, in my experience, never questioned or contradicted. If something was necessary but unavailable, the hospital administration got it. And, being a municipal hospital, all nonclinical paperwork was handled by the hospital. Computers had arrived, but, except for technical and laboratory applications and reports, were still somewhat a mystery on the wards. As clinicians, we on the staff could still concentrate on the important issues for which we were trained.

With the preceding as a statement on present and pending issues for our medical profession, an overview of the history of medical practice in prior civilizations may provide insight into what may happen if things do not change. The issues, conclusions and recommendations are of a general nature and oriented toward the role of centralized governance in the provision of medical care. They are not intended to stop analytic discourse on a sensitive issue. In fact, such discourse should increase. But hopefully it will be local, it will be diverse, and it will provide more solutions to present-day problems because it will move out of the dark shadow of an overweening government that stacks the deck on open deliberation and prevents, sometimes by criminalizing, opposing views. This aim, through the study of the history of medical practice, has been previously stated:

ζητειν αὐτῆς μὲν τὴν γένεσεν, ἦν δὲ δύνωμαι,
ἀποδιδόναι δὲ ἀνθρώπῳ τέχνην τὴν ἰατρικήν.
"To seek its origin and, if I can,
Return the art of medicine to man."
Anonymous Fragment[3]

Medical progress as documented in ancient civilizations

To begin this excursus, here are several corollaries that I claim support the notion that all medical progress is traceable to the physician-patient relation.

---

[3] See title page, volume 1, of *The Natural State of Medical Practice: An Isagorial Theory of Human Progress*, Liberty Hill Press, 2019.

1. All human societies have equivalent and broadly distributed intellectual potential, regardless of race, ethnicity or chronological era. This extends back tens of thousands of years to the upper Paleolithic. The idea that intrinsic human intellectual potential has increased since the Stone Age is absurd.
2. All humans and human societies have equivalent motivation for seeking and developing effective medical care because disease, trauma, pain and death equally afflict persons of all ages and stations of life.
3. Initiation of medical progress is simple, easy, cheap, readily available, and requires no technology. We call it the medical history and physical examination.
4. The best objective measure we have of a civilization's progress is life expectancy for the unprivileged classes. Art, literature, and displays of wealth of an elite political class are more a reflection of its degree of authoritarianism than evidence of progress, our own civilization excepted for reasons to be discussed later.

For anyone who strongly disagrees with any of these points, the following discussion will probably be of little interest.

Given equal range of intellectual potential in all human societies, ancient and modern, a specialty that is quick, easy, simple, convenient and cheap in its acquisition of knowledge, and equal susceptibility to factors driving motivation to lessen pain, restore health, and prevent death, medicine as a profession should have been among the first specialties to be devised within human society and among the first to be improved with passage of time, *i.e.*, to progress. As described in *The Natural State of Medical Practice*, it should have popped up in early civilizations, and so it did.

Evidence of early rational medicine is found in five ancient medical treatises that are acclaimed by regional scholars as fundamental classics of their respective civilizations and are dated to their early years. Extent representatives of the five are:[4]

---

[4] Evidence of rational medical practices is widely cited, prominent assessments including the following: (1) Scurlock, J., and Andersen, B., *Diagnoses in Assyrian and Babylonian Medicine: Ancient Sources, Translations, and Modern Medical Analyses*, Urbana, 2005; (2) Ghaliougui, P., *The Ebers Papyrus: A New Translation, Commentaries and Glossaries*, Cairo, 1987; and Majno, G., *The Healing Hand*, Cambridge (MA), 1975, chapter 3; (3) the prominent scholar, Dr. A. C. Kaviratna, described the Charaka Samhita, which he translated, as "the greatest scientific work of ancient Indian wisdom," the Encyclopedia Britannica characterizes the Charaka Samhita as the "encyclopedia of Ayurvedic medicine," and B. Patwardhan, *Bridging Auurveda with Evidence-based Scientific Approaches to Medicine*, in *EPMA Journal* 5:19, 2014; (4) Unschuld, P. U., *Huang Di Nei Jing Su Wen*, Berkeley, 2003, and (5) John Chadwick and W. H. Mann, MD, FRCP, *The Medical Works of Hippocrates*, Illinois, 1950. Fairly consistent dating is present only for the Hippocratic Corpus. Dating of the others varies considerably, and the supporting evidence for the dates given herein is presented in *The Natural State of Medical Practice*, vols. 1 and 3. Furthermore, collection of data on which these treatises were based necessarily had to begin one or two centuries earlier.

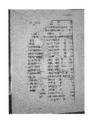 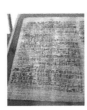 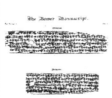 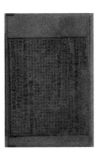 

Left to right:

1. Representing Sumer, the *Treatise of Medical Diagnosis and Prognosis* (*ca.* 3000 BC) is Labat's copy of a forty clay tablet 7th C BC version of an edited 11th C BC Babylonian version of the *Treatise* containing elements of ancient Sumerian wisdom

2. Egyptian papyri, primarily *Papyrus Ebers* (*ca.* 3000 BC, but this is the earliest extant copy of 1530 BC)

3. *Charaka Samhita* ("The Collection of Charaka") (*ca.* 2000 BC); no early copies; this is the earliest extant partial copy on birch bark of the related *Susruta Samhita* from the 6th C AD

4. *Huang Ti Nei Ching Su Wen* (*The Yellow Emperor's Classic of Internal Medicine*; Veith's translation) (*ca.* 2400 BC); oldest copy (edited in 8th C AD by Wang Bing) is from the 17th C AD

5. *Corpus Hippocraticum* (5th century BC); fragment of the Hippocratic Oath, 2nd C AD

The proposed dates of the earliest appearance of these five medical writings are unavoidably estimates as none of the originals exist and some may have been orally transmitted prior to collation into a single document. But, based on both objective and circumstantial evidence, the proposed dates when the initial clinical observations were made are supported by reasonable argument as presented in *The Natural State of Medical Practice*, vol. 3. There will be disagreement on this point, but there is no question that all are ancient and from the early years of their respective civilizations. By the dates given, note that all but the *Corpus Hippocraticum* border on the Neolithic in their origin, the Greek appearing during the late Archaic period (*ca.* 600-500 BC), perhaps in the city of Miletus that was founded *de novo* in 1050 BC by a presumably migratory Hellenic population. Acute and thoughtful clinical observations are present in all five treatises, examples being given in *The Natural State of Medical Practice*, vols. 1 and 2.

It is also proposed that medical progress can be considered a surrogate for estimating progress in general, and my broad definition of "progress" is:

PROGRESS: A social concept based on the **awareness of improvability** of the human condition.

It has been stated that medicine in ancient Greece was considered the only truly scientific intellectual discipline and that its success was a stimulus to progress in other areas.[5]

---

[5] This, in fact, was the opinion of Hippocrates: "I also hold that clear knowledge about natural science can be acquired from medicine and from no other source." (*Ancient Medicine*, XX, translation of W. H. S. Jones). The reason for this seemingly pretentious statement is that

Physician and patient: the foundation of all medical progress

It was mentioned earlier that medical progress is simple, easy, cheap, readily available and requires no technology. This, of course, is a description of the medical history and physical examination of a patient. To support this claim, here are a few examples by physicians of the recent past, none of whom were from privileged families and none whose invention required Einsteinian genius, who have been hailed as founders of modern medicine:

1. Morgagni's classic work

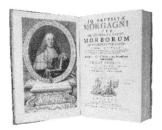

Dr. Giovanni Battista Morgagni (1682-1771) at the age of eighty published his *De Sedibus et Causis Morborum per Anatomen Indagatus* (Venice, 1761), a classic in medical literature that correlated, in hundreds of individual cases, careful autopsy findings with clinical signs and symptoms. As a professor at the medical school in Padua for sixty years he maintained careful notes of all his work, but his major publication was done late in life at the advice of a friend. He thus moved anatomy from the realm of the descriptive and passive to the dynamic. There had been earlier studies of anatomic pathology, for the brother of Antonio Benivieni (1440-1502) published Antonio's results of one hundred and eleven autopsies in 1507 (*De Abditis nonn ulis ac mirandis Morborum et Sanationum Causis*), but the purpose of those autopsies was more for anatomical study than clinical relevance. **It was Dr. Morgagni's association of clinical status of many patients with autopsy findings of specific diseased organs that moved medicine into the modern age**.

2. Auenbrugger's invention

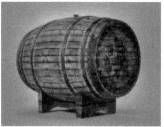

Inspiration for percussion: checking level of wine in barrels.

Hippocratic medicine was the only objective discipline within the framework of ancient Greek natural philosophy.

Dr. Leopold Auenbrugger (1722-1809) is credited with the invention of the technique of percussion. This clinical tool must have been familiar to the Ancients, although its first known descriptions are by Aretaeus (1st C AD) and then by Alexander of Tralles in the 6th C AD. Thereafter it seems to have been forgotten, although percussion of the cranium of sheep was used by 17th C shepherds to diagnose hydatid cysts, as noted by Dr. van Swieten. But modern concepts of percussion can be traced to Dr. Auenbrugger who described a method of tapping on the surface of the body in such a way that the subsurface density could be estimated.[6] As a child he had watched his father, an innkeeper, tap on the sides of wine casks to determine their fullness. In 1753, after becoming a physician, he applied the same method to examination of the chest and found he could differentiate consolidation, effusion, and pneumothorax by carefully assessing the sound and tactile vibration produced by the tapping on the chest wall. After seven years of correlating percussion findings with clinical course, surgery, or autopsy findings, he published, in Latin, a ninety-five-page description in 1761. Dr. Auenbrugger acknowledged no other description or work on percussion antedating his discovery. He said it was "new." But what made Dr. Auenbrugger's invention monumental was his correlation of percussion results with clinical status, surgical and post-mortem findings, and related observations, and then publishing his analysis. The importance of the clinician's touch in turning a device or procedure, simple or complex, into a touchstone for medical science should now be apparent. It can be stated, in fact, that **it was the inventing clinician's attention to his patients more than his invention that was the great event,** a sequence that led to many a famous physician's prominence and one that was readily available in ancient, classical and modern times.

3.   Laennec's invention

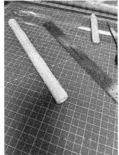 Rolled up quire of paper, the first stethoscope

Dr. Rene Laennec (1781-1826) invented indirect, or mediate, auscultation with his version of the stethoscope. Direct auscultation (*e.g.*, ear on the chest) had been the standard procedure for at least 2300 years. Dr. Laennec cited Hippocratic observations on succussion in his epochal publication in 1819, but they were not the stimulus for his discovery. In 1816, desiring to listen to the chest in an overweight young woman with heart disease, he recalled "the augmented impression of sound when conveyed through

---

[6] Auenbrugger, L., *Inventum Novum ex Percussione Thoracis Humani ut Signo Abstrusos Interni Pectoris Morbos Detegendi* (New Invention to Detect Diseases Hidden Deep Inside the Chest), Vienna, 1761, the translator of the English version, *On Percussion of the Chest* (London, 1824) being John Forbes..

certain solid bodies, - as when we hear the scratch of a pin at one end of a piece of wood, on applying our ear to the other." He reached for a rolled-up quire of paper (see Figure). He found her heart sounds more distinct than usually heard when placing the ear directly against the chest, and at the same time he avoided embarrassment to his patient.[7] The invention was, however, not solid wood. It was a tube, and at the distal end there was a wooden stopper, and with this in place he could better hear the heart sounds and variations in transmission of the voice, whereas with the plug removed it was the breath sounds that were clearer.[8] Importantly, there was no evolution in technique of auscultation between the time of the Hippocratics and Laennec that made the invention of the stethoscope more likely to be his discovery than theirs. And yet many of the diagnoses by stethoscope could also have been made by placing the ear directly on the affected and surrounding area. The usefulness of direct auscultation is shown by the fact that some clinicians were slow to accept Laennec's invention because they did not view it as a significant improvement, and certain benefits of "immediate" auscultation have been recently pointed out.[9] **The critical component of Dr. Laennec's work was not so much his invention, although it was an improvement over "immediate" auscultation. It was, instead, his acute clinical description of chest and heart sounds in relation to symptoms, other signs, clinical outcome, and internal anatomy as detected at post-mortem examination or surgical procedure that made his work immortal.**

---

[7] Laennec, R. T. H., *A Treatise on the Diseases of the Chest*, London, 1821, translated by J. Forbes, MD, p. 281*ff*. The original was *De l'Auscultation Mediate*, Paris, 1819.

[8] The concentration of sound by means of the ear trumpet might have suggested to someone a way to improve on direct auscultation, for cupping one's hand behind the ear to improve auditory acuity is no modern discovery. Instruments for improving auditory acuity over great distances have an ancient history among mariners, and ear trumpets were first mentioned in 1624. Kircher determined that a megaphone of sufficient size could carry a voice for several miles. Improvements on the stethoscope would include its evolution into an instrument that relies solely on transmitting amplified sound waves via air through tubing. Jean Leurechon (Henrik van Etten, *Recreations Mathematiques*, sixth edition, Lyon, 1627) describes the use of tubes to conduct sound for purposes of overhearing conversations of others (Problem 59). The Leurechon work also displays an engraving of an early thermometer.

[9] Puddu, V., *Immediate Auscultation – An Old Method Not to be Forgotten*, in *Circulation*, 52:526-527, 1975.

4. Pare's classic work (1585)

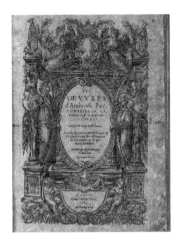

The barber-surgeon, Ambroise Pare (1510-1590), in 1549 published an anatomical work that included a description of internal podalic version. Pare acknowledged that he learned of the technique not from familiarity with ancient writings but from discussions with two other Parisian barber-surgeons who were using it and who learned it from local midwives.[10] Soranus, 2nd C AD Greek physician and author of the most credible life of Hippocrates, had also wonderfully described the procedure. **It was, therefore, not Pare's "invention" of podalic version that added to his fame, for it had already been invented. But as an accomplished surgeon it was his published description of the technique based on his personal clinical experience with it in obstetric patients** that was now available for other physicians to see. His candid statement regarding the source of the technique is a peek into the unwritten history of mankind, for rediscovery of the obviously important is the natural way of things. The tendency to associate an important discovery with a singular individual subsequently declared to be a person superior in one way or another ignores the work of innumerable other discoverers of whom nothing is ever to be known. Another example follows.

5. Withering's foxglove, source of digitalis

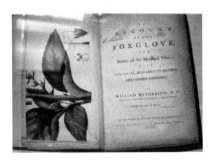

---

[10] The two other barber-surgeons, friends of Pare, were Thierry de Hery and Nicole Lambert, the latter his godfather, as cited in Dr. Francis Packard's *The Life and Times of Ambrose Pare*, New York, 1921, a publication which includes Packard's translations of some of Pare's works.

Dr. William Withering (1741-1799) identified an active principle by isolating the leaves of *Digitalis purpurea* from a mixture of herbs mentioned to him by an elderly woman in Shropshire, an herbalist. **From his observations on his patients he confirmed the usefulness of the foxglove and determined the optimal preparation to be administered, along with quantifying effective and toxic doses.** Squill is another botanical containing cardiac glycosides and it was used for dropsy by the ancients and into the 18th C. The value of cardiac glycosides in treating "dropsy" is found in their ability to improve heart function and/or rhythm and rate. The generic term, digitalis, has been applied to the cardioactive principal in foxglove, and for almost two hundred years "digitalis" in various forms was a mainstay in cardiac care.[11]

6.   An axillary thermometer

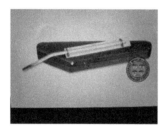

Dr. Carl Wunderlich (1815-1877) is credited for clinical relevance of the thermometer. He was aware of experiments in the development of the thermometer at the University in Padua, where Galileo and others exploited the knowledge exposed by the recent publication, after some 1500 years, of the writings of the 1st C AD Greek mathematician, Hero, in matters dealing with air pressure and siphons.[12]   Several successful demonstrations of early thermometers had occurred since the 17th C, but the "fever hospital" in London in 1830 had no thermometers. The pivotal event relevant to the thermometer can be ascribed to Dr. Wunderlich who, in 1868, reported accurate serial temperature measurements in 25,000 episodes of febrile illness, and from his millions of observations using an axillary thermometer a valuable fine tuning of determining body temperature became widely popular.[13] The practiced hand can distinguish among no, low,

---

[11] A recent recounting of the discovery of foxglove as an herbal therapy and an admission that the name of the Shropshire woman who successfully used it remains unknown is found in: Kahn, R. J., *William Withering's Wonderful Weed*, in *Clio in the Clinic: History in Medical Practice*, Oxford, 2005, J. Duffin, editor, pp. 189-200. Powdered digitalis leaf, in a standardized dose, was used to treat Winston Churchill in 1943, and it was in the Bellevue Hospital formulary, 100 mg tablets, when I interned there in 1962.

[12] The *Pneumatica* of Hero of Alexandria was published first in Italian in Bologna (1547). The more widely read Latin version was published in 1575. Galileo's dates are 1564-1642, so Hero's ideas would have been available to him. Also to be considered as inventor of the thermometer is Philo of Byzantium (280-220 BC), from whom Hero of Alexandria may have received the idea of heating causing expansion of gas volume.

[13] Wunderlich, C. A., *On the Temperature in Diseases*, a publication of the New Sydenham Society, London, 1871, translated from the German by W. B. Woodman. Chapter II gives an exhaustive history of the development of the thermometer. It is a measure of the wide acceptance and obvious great value of Wunderlich's studies that the Sydenham Society, which published classics such as translations of Hippocrates and Aretaeus, chose to print in its entirety a translation of Wunderlich's

moderate, or high fever if care is taken to adjust for cutaneous vasoconstriction and other variables. For many patients this alone can be adequate in diagnosis and treatment. The clinical value of the thermometer lies as much in the ease of repeated measurements as in its precision, although it does away with interobserver variability. Dr. Wunderlich went on to describe the utility of graphed values. But if he had personally assessed by hand every four hours or so the fevers of all his 25,000 patients and correlated the graphed results with clinical outcome, the quality of the data, while distinctly inferior to those obtained with a thermometer, would still have been of great clinical value to the profession and therefore to patients. **Without clinical correlations the clinical thermometer has no value, and clinical relevance was what Dr. Wunderlich provided.**

7. Semmelweis' classic work

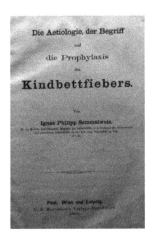

Dr. Joseph Lister (1827-1912) published his famous paper in *The Lancet* in 1865-67 describing the practical control of puerperal fever with carbolic acid. Dr. Alexander Gordon had, in 1795, published a book in which he clearly explained the epidemiology and control of puerperal sepsis, and Dr. Oliver Wendell Holmes had popularized the danger of contagion in 1843, later published in 1855 (Boston) in a book called *Puerperal Fever*. The data were not his own, instead being his clinical interpretation of reports on childbed fever from around the world. Dr. Ignaz Semmelweis published his first clinical report on prevention of childbed fever in 1858. The purpose of this extensive commentary is, in part, to provide evidence that a journal was more effective in disseminating professional information than was a book, but also to point out that criticism of Semmelweis' work from some European sources greatly impeded acceptance of his recommendations. This sad state of affairs has been attributed, rightly, to an authoritarian legacy apparent in Dr. Rudolph Virchow and many other prominent 19th C magisterial professors. J. H. Baas, in his *Outlines of the History of Medicine and the Medical Profession* (New York, 1889, H. E. Handerson, translator, p. 1083), has perfectly described the process: "... the discoverers of truth now are no longer crucified, but their names are simply written upon the proscription-list of the *lease-holders of science*" (italics

---

work only three years after its first appearance in German (*Das Verhalten der Eigenwarme in Krankheiten*, Leipzig, 1868).

added). Lease-holders of science were, gratefully up to the early 20th C, least evident in America. Today, of course, the lease-holder of science has reemerged: big government.

8. 6th C BC quartz lenses, Rhodes Museum of Archeology

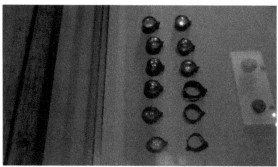

Magnifying lenses were available for making jewelry in the 6th C BC. In a sense the preceding vignettes are similar to the situation with magnifying lenses; the important 19th C advances in magnification, in measurement of body temperature, listening to heart sounds, detecting shifting dullness, and in other areas, were due to clinical application rather than just discovery or rediscovery. It was the clinician's elaboration on and use of discoveries that determined a discovery's value. Regarding the lenses, some had magnification power sufficient to see blood flowing through capillaries. It is likely, therefore, that similar elaboration on and use of those same discoveries, including microscopic analysis, would have been successfully undertaken by Hippocratic physicians given a bit more time.

From the preceding examples it can be concluded that it is clinical observation by the physician, and the clinical physician alone, that is the initiating source of medical progress. It is physicians' attentiveness to their patients that is the basis for disease identification and taxonomy, the stimulus for all research for therapies, procedures, and instrumentation, and clinical basis for both personal advice and epidemiological and public policies. It is the physicians' attentiveness to their patients that provides the evidence that justifies, or not, the safety and usefulness of innovative ideas. The intellectual arena in which the physician functions is shared by no one else, just as with any profession, and it follows that only physicians can judge the quality of the process and the final product. When this arena is compromised by those outside the profession or when a physician is directed to do something that is unwarranted or unnecessary in patient care by policies devised by those outside the profession, the usefulness, the credibility and the reputation of physicians is damaged.

The ancient Greeks knew all this to be true. Hippocratic physicians were not spokesmen for the local city-state tyrant or governing council. There might be complaints, but, as Plato put it, "We believe in them [doctors] whether they cure us with our consent or without it,[...]." [14] As per Plato, the source of the physician's authority is

---

[14] Plato's *Statesman*, 293b, translation of C. J. Rowe, in *Plato; Complete Works*, Indianapolis, 1997, J. M. Cooper, editor. This matter is discussed by G. Anagnastopoulos in: *Bioethics: Ancient Themes in Contemporary Issues*, Boston, 2002 (paperback edition), M. G. Kuczewski and R. Polansky, editors, p. 279*ff*.

rather blatant; there is no one else who knows medicine better than the physician, so the matter is ended. He stated that if there were a medical legal challenge, it was only other physicians who could pass judgment.[15]

From progress to regress

Four of the five ancient civilizations mentioned earlier did not progress further in medicine. Their ancient medical texts, containing knowledge acquired in the early phases of their respective civilizations, therefore represented their equivalent of Harrison's *Principles of Internal Medicine*, except that Harrison's is now in its 21st edition in only seventy years, whereas there was no "second edition" of any of the ancient works over thousands of years, although some editing and amendments occurred. They did not continue to progress, and sometimes they regressed:

(1) Mesopotamia: Despite the early medical discoveries in Sumer (*ca.* 3000 BC, although mature cuneiform writing would not be available for three centuries) and their editing by the non-physician, Esagil-kin-apli, in the 11th C BC, Herodotus visited Babylonia in the 5th C BC and described the situation thus:

"I come now to the next wisest of their customs: having no use for physicians, they carry the sick into the market-place; then those who have been afflicted themselves by the same ill as the sick man's, or seen others in like case, come near and advise him about his disease and comfort him, telling him by what means they have themselves recovered of it or seen others so recover."

After two thousand years, plenty of time for professional associations to improve, he identified no medical practitioners at all.

(2) Egypt: The eminent physician and historian of medicine, Dr. John Nunn, concluded:

"There is no evidence of major changes in the format or content of classical Egyptian medicine between the old kingdom and the end of the Twenty-sixth Dynasty, covering the years 2600 to 525 BC. This may be inscribed to the innate conservatism of the Egyptians, ..."[16]

(3) India: Dr. Debiprasad Chattopadhyaya, eminent philosopher and historian of science who described early medical writings in India as indicating a belief in causality, that a disease was an entity rather than a status, and that curability could reside in the actions of a physician, considered them of great importance despite "the heap of intellectual debris eventually dumped on them" as they were subsumed by Hinduism's Brahmin caste.[17] Regarding the *Charaka Samhita*, his praise was reserved only for its earliest content.

---

[15] See Plato's *Nomoi* (Laws), 916 a-c.
[16] Nunn, J. F., *Ancient Egyptian Medicine*, London, 1996, p. 206.
[17] See Dr. Chattopadhyaya's excellent book, *Science and Society in Ancient India* (Bangalore, 1977) for an explication of this topic.

(4) China: Lastly, consider the observation of Prof. Sivin, a prominent historian and Sinologist, regarding the course of Chinese medicine:

"The classics are documents of the scholarly traditions that developed on the edges of the small, literate, office-holding elite, and which treated few of those outside it (and few of its women)."[18]   More relevant here is his observation that: "We know practically nothing about the practitioners who could not be called physicians… who actually were the peasant majority's only source of therapy."[19]

(5) The Greek, or the Greco-Roman, civilization was different. Hippocratic medicine was allowed two centuries to evolve, with a few discoveries as late as the 3rd C BC. Then, in a civilization smitten by authoritarian wars and Roman conquest, it merely vanished like a journal that is not renewed. This was followed by absence of progress for 1500 years through the Dark Ages and medieval Europe.

That something so simple and basic, something that was recognized as helping everyone, did not develop further in these civilizations, a negating social factor of considerable magnitude must have been involved in the successive dynasties of these four civilizations. If those civilizations did not progress in medicine, did they progress in other areas?

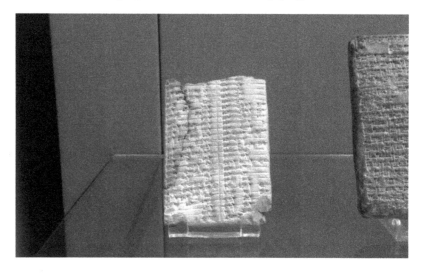

(1) A bilingual clay tablet, Mesopotamia

The forceful unification of the Sumerian aggregate of city-states (2350 BC) was followed by a sequence of totalitarian dynasties, including Akkadian, Amorite, Kassite, Babylonian and Assyrian and Persian (559-330 BC). The importance of the early advances in medicine, mathematics and other technical fields is

---

[18] See the review by Dr. Nathan Sivin in: *Social History of Medicine,* 19:334-336, 2006, p. 336.
[19] Sivin, N., his Introduction to volume 6, part VI, of the classic series *Science and Civilization in China*, by Needham, J., and Gwei-Djen, L., Cambridge, 2004, p. 195, footnote.

reflected in the retention of the Sumerian cuneiform text through subsequent empires (even to the 4th C BC) and, in some cases, a panoramic rather than portrait shape to clay tablets, often, as in the photograph, side-by-side with the contemporary cuneiform version (*e.g.*, Akkadian, Babylonian). In contrast, in other areas such as literature and bureaucratic writings, only the contemporary cuneiform was used. The desire to retain this anchor to past wisdom suggests there was not much new wisdom with which to replace or improve it.

(2) Narmer palette and pyramidion Wedjahol, Egypt; each about two feet tall, but the Narmer palette on the left is 3,000 years older. Art similar, quality worse.

[

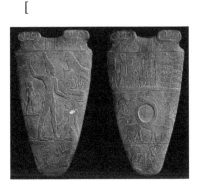 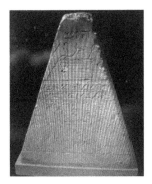

Over a sequence of almost 30 dynasties there was remarkably little change in Egyptian art. Diodorus Siculus (1st C BC) wrote:

"Since the Egyptian artist had no idea of perspective, each part of a figure, or each member of a group, was portrayed as if seen from directly in front. Therefore, the first training of the artist consisted in the making of the separate members of the body, which accounts for the many heads, hands, legs, and feet, which come from the Egyptian schools of art."

The role of the State in defining art is obvious. Canonization of art was mirrored in the canonization of medical practice.

(3) Ruins of Mohenjo Daro, ancient India

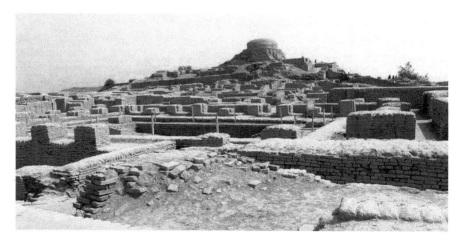

It is impossible to discern evidence of progress in the subcontinent inasmuch as there was a dispersion of monarchical centers throughout the subcontinent following the disintegration of the remarkable Indus River Valley Civilization that began *ca.* 2000 BC.[20] There was no major city prior to that of Pataliputra in the 4th C BC when it became the center of the vast Mauryan empire. In contrast to the relatively egalitarian Indus River Valley city of Mohenjo Daro, Pataliputra had a large palace and there is no mention of sewage disposal other than a large ditch on the city's periphery, whereas most dwellings in Mohenjo Daro had in-house toilets served by city-wide system of covered sewers, bricks indicated standardized production, and the layout of the city was planned. Of the two cities, only ancient Mohenjo Daro with its apparent absence of a political hierarchy suggests progress.

(4) Han compass, 1st C BC, China

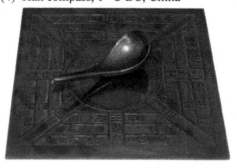

---

[20] Present scholarly opinion is that weather change underlay the decline of the Indus River Valley Civilization. It is conceivable that the seemingly advanced status of the city of Mohenjo Daro in the civilization was in an advanced settlement hierarchy phase of development, perhaps similar to that of Uruk before the Mesopotamian dynastic age.

It is one of the mysteries of Chinese inventions that rarely did one succeed in becoming socially beneficial. Dr. Joseph Needham identified some 271 inventions that followed this pattern.[21] As for printing, Chinese characters, which number in tens of thousands, pose a significant difficulty for moveable type, and this probably made it impractical for extensive medical texts to be printed until recent times.

(5) The West:

The progress of mathematics has been mirrored in the frequency of major advances and their inventors. One authoritative book lists on its endpapers, from 600 BC to 400 AD there were nine prominent mathematicians, and from 1400 to 1900 there were seventeen. During the intervening period there were none.

Although more data and analyses of other specializations are desired, **it is a reasonable postulate that societal progress in general mirrors medical progress**.

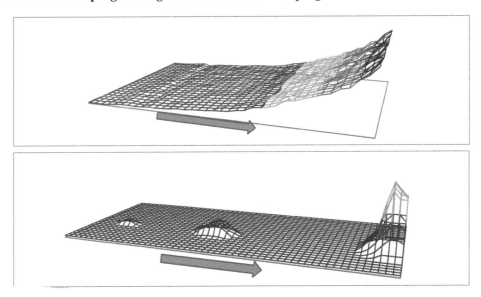

Above are two postulated graphs of medical progress in the history civilizations. To summarize these figures, the top figure represents the popular conception of human progress, namely that we continue to build on our predecessors' knowledge as it accumulates throughout the world. There is no turning back, no regression. Sadly, this is incorrect. The bottom figure shows how a civilization returns to its empiric baseline when progress is arrested by authoritarian political hierarchies. The small blips on the

---

[21] For the reasons, see: Lowrey, Y. and Baumol, W. J., *Rapid Invention, Slow Industrialization, and the Absent Innovative Entrepreneur in Medieval China*, a paper read at a meeting of the American Economic Association, Atlanta, Jan. 3-5, 2010, and for "the Needham puzzle" see Lin, J. Y., *The Needham Puzzle: Why the Industrial Revolution did not originate in China*, in *Economic Development and Cultural Change*, 43:269-292, 1995.

left side of the bottom graph represent nascent medical progress as documented in the ancient medical writings 4000-5000 years ago, but authoritarianism usurped management of medical care. In India it was canonized and under control of the Brahmans of the Hindu caste system, in Egypt it was canonized and subsumed by Pharaonic priests, in China it was canonized and relegated to the elite kinships, and in Mesopotamia it was replaced by mysticism.

Greece, the middle blip, was different in that its medical progress declined with the disintegration of society followed by the Roman conquest 2200 years ago. Hippocratic physicians were left alone; they just disappeared because the plebeian population, given the social environment, was unable to carry on the Greek medical tradition. At the same time, alternative therapies became popular. But Hippocratic medicine persisted unimpeded sufficiently long to have a prominent legacy.

The largest blip is our own. Compared to the others it is massive in size and somewhat longer in duration. Its onset is set at the Reformation (500 years ago), for reasons discussed elsewhere. I have designed it showing we are now on the downward slope. The reason for this interpretation will be touched on later, but the greater significance for the downward trend of all the portrayed civilizations is the basis for this excursus.

Cessation of medical progress; its cause

Initiation of ancient medical progress can be dated roughly to a stage in early urbanization of "primary" city-states known as the "settlement hierarchy." Archeologists define this as:

> SETTLEMENT HIERARCHY: A natural progression of intergroup adjustments that spontaneously occurs as an urbanizing society, having no prior experience with a political hierarchy, becomes more complex and acquires facilities, goods and services to accommodate an enlarging population.

The settlement hierarchy and its progress ended with the appearance of centralized authoritarian political domination of the early city-states that would grow to become empires. The cessation of medical progress was not because of dislike of medical practitioners and their knowledge. Practitioners came from general population and were no threat to the powerful. In fact, the privileged class generally viewed them as useful, the ancient Egyptians and Chinese dynasties incorporating them into their elite political hierarchy, Chinese monarchs even periodically commanding the collection and publication of encyclopedic editions of medicinals from practitioners around their country.

As there was no hostility by governance directed at the humble practitioner, for reasons to be discussed later it is proposed that canonization of medicine was an important reason for cessation of progress and that canonization was a policy originating from the political hierarchy. Did any of the five civilizations identify strongly with canonization?

(1) Egypt – Diodorus Siculus made the following statement on Egyptian medicine in the 1st C BC. It reveals the reverence felt for canonical medical practices and the penalty for sceptics:

"On their military campaigns and their journeys in the country they all receive treatment without the payment of any private fee; for the physicians draw their support from public funds and administer their treatments in accordance with a written law which was composed in ancient times by many famous physicians. **If they follow the rules of this law as they read them in the sacred book and yet are unable to save their patient, they are absolved from any charge and go unpunished; but if they go contrary to the law's prescriptions in any respect, they must submit to a trial with death as the penalty**, the lawgiver holding that but few physicians would ever show themselves wiser than the mode of treatment which had been closely followed for a long period and had been originally prescribed by the ablest practitioners."[22]

Ancient Egyptian physicians within two or three dynasties after unification of Egypt (3100 BC) had become a pharaonic factotum, they and their knowledge canonized for 2500 years.

(2) China – Confucius in the 6th C BC was able to recognize "a good physician" as distinct from a magician.[23] By the 4th C BC medical practitioners considered satisfactory for the elite class were beginning to be acquired by integrating Confucian concepts into the examination system used to ensure a compliant civil service for the elite class. Thus, the chosen medical professionals were philosophically sympathetic to the authoritarian State and dedicated to the dynastic leadership.[24] Once chosen, medical outcomes determined advancement. The profound significance of the Confucian canon in Chinese history is conveniently presented by Prof. Thomas A. Wilson.[25] Ancient Chinese physicians during the subsequent Han dynasty (206 BC) had become little more than State employees serving the ruling class, their knowledge fixed in time. That knowledge was the already ancient knowledge of the *Huang Ti Nei Ching Su Wen.*

(3) India - The knowledge of the early rational practitioners became, or was from the beginning, oral tradition, but with the evolution of Hinduism the Brahman elite class "piled a heap of intellectual debris" on that rational knowledge and took over the training of practitioners as a written form of Sanskrit came into use. It is stated that Manu, the giver of laws, prohibited high-caste Hindus from accepting any food from physicians because that food "is like pus and blood." Edited knowledge of the *Charaka Samhita* is traced to Charaka, postulated to be a Hindu physician of the 1st C BC who was canonized as an archetypical physician, and the source of the knowledge he is supposed to have collated was

---

[22] *Diodorus Siculus*, Bk. I, 82, 3, the *Loeb Classical Library* translation of C. H. Oldfather. A notable feature of this passage is absence of the concept of progress, for it indicates that perfection in medicine was considered to have been reached 2,500 years earlier, and to attempt any improvement was perilous, a comment not on the medicine but on ancient Egyptian governance.

[23] Mentioned by Joseph Needham and Lu Gwei-Djen in *Medicine and Culture*, London, 1969, p. 256.

[24] See: Dien, A. E., *State and Society in Early Medieval China*, Stanford, 1990. Also, Dr. Majno, referenced earlier, comments on the status of Confucianism, pointing out the contemporary good opinion of physicians.

[25] See website of "Cult of Confucius." Under the aegis of Prof. Thomas A. Wilson of Hamilton College, Clinton, NY, the remarkable long and effective canonization of Confucius is displayed. academics.hamilton.edu/asian_studies/home/culttemp/index.html

further canonized by being attributed to mythical/legendary figures, including Agnivesa and the Hindu sage, Atreya. The ancient Indian practitioner would remain fixed in time.

(4) Mesopotamia - Mysticism, made prominent during the Akkadian subjugation of Sumer (2350 BC), superseded the rational practitioner, the *azu*. The latter had become regulated by the State (Code of Ur-Nammu). Hammurabi then listed on his famous stele in 1750 BC the penalties that would be brought to bear on the *azu* should there be an unsatisfactory surgical outcome (see below).[26] Sumerian medical writing was nevertheless canonized, and later editings superimposed strong elements of magic. Even the prominent *Treatise of Medical Diagnosis and Prognosis* as it was edited in the 11th C BC was actually addressed to the practitioners of magic (the *asipu*) even though much content was rational medical knowledge of the early Sumerian *azu*. Thus, canonization of rational medicine was placed in the hands of the newly canonized practitioner, the *asipu* (the sorcerer priest). The sorcerer priest was not going to risk his career with medical innovation, and the Mesopotamian practitioner (*azu*) for some time disappeared altogether.

From the Code of Hammurabi:
P218 – If a physician performs major surgery with a bronze lancet upon an ...... and thus causes the .....'s death, or opens an ......'s temple with a bronze lancet and thus blinds the ......'s eye, they shall cut off his hand.
P219 – If a physician performs major surgery with a bronze lancet upon a slave of a commoner and thus causes the slave's death, he shall replace the slave with a slave of comparable value.
P220 – If he opens his (the commoner's slave's) temple with a bronze lancet and thus blinds his eye, he shall weigh and deliver silver equal to half his value.

(5) Ancient Greece - Hippocratic treatises were not canonized by any contemporary elite class. Canonization occurred later. In the Middle East, and Avicenna wrote his treatise on medicine (1025 AD), its translated title being *The Canon of Medicine*, much of it Hippocratic, which Dr. William Osler declared the "most famous medical text ever written." And in the Late Medieval Period, "physicians" in the medieval guilds and the evolving university systems admired and taught the words of Hippocrates but not Hippocratic methods. Hippocrates and his medical writings were canonized and would remain unaltered and unimproved.

It is reasonable to conclude that the cessation or loss of early medical knowledge was a consequence of authoritarian policies which tended to canonize both the author(s) and the medical knowledge itself, thus making it refractory to change and ineligible for progress. As for those early physicians who were the initial source of the rational medical knowledge found in the medical classics of their respective civilizations, after perhaps one or two centuries only limited remnants of their knowledge survived to be assembled or reassembled by subsequent compilers and editors, the *Hippocratic Corpus* excepted.

---

[26] The selected laws are from *The Letters and Inscription of Hammurabi, King of Babylon, about B. C. 2200*, London, 1898, translated by L. W. King.

Relevance to modern American medicine

Without exception, all governments inevitably seek greater power, but the American Constitution and Bill of Rights have provided a firewall against this reflex. The federal government in the past century, however, has been actively pursuing the goals and applying tactics similar to those employed by authoritarian governments of the past. In a modern version, it increasingly directs medical training, medical research, and medical practice based on political relevance, arguing that expert opinion is being followed. Like the ancient Akkadians, it is creating *de facto* seers, a few select experts whom it considers more knowledgeable than everyone else, just as the ancient Akkadians embraced their mystic, the *asipu*. Today it also is a prominent few, often with limited clinical experience, that guide a national health policy, and the individual practitioner who knows that every patient is unique in expression of disease is being pressured into compliance. To expedite the spread of that policy, like the Pharaohs, government increasingly entangles and integrates practitioners and their organizations into its operations. Just like ancient China and Confucianism, it supports medical practitioners politically sympathetic to the social goals of government.

In government hands, medicine becomes but another political tool, with the practitioner's loyalty subtly shifted from the patient to the agency. How can American medicine be adversely affected by canonization, complicity (corporatism), incompetence, and destabilization emanating from government?

Canonization:

The breadth and depth of medical knowledge is vast. Overall there is no possibility of canonization of the bulk of that knowledge, for it is in so many hands, collegially divided among so many different practitioners, and changes and updates frequently. Unlike ancient civilizations, there is no core clinical treatise that can be considered essential to medical practice to which all can be made to adhere. But that is not the whole story.

The term "canon" is distantly derived from the Greek κανῶν, meaning a rule or straight-edge that precisely defines a boundary or distinction. The Oxford English Dictionary makes clear its authoritative nature as its synonyms "law, rule, edict" imply. Aspects of canonization include:

1. Canonization of knowledge – The texts or proposed sources of the classic medical manuscripts were canonized as subsequent dynasties referred to their ancient sources with reverence and deferred to their wisdom (*Argumentum ad Verecundiam*). Rote acceptance of prior medical knowledge was prominent in earlier civilizations as if that knowledge had been and would remain the gold standard for medical practice. The concept of improvement over time, *i.e.*, progress, was not a consideration. This was also the European perspective on Hippocratic writings as it emerged from the Dark Ages but is not an issue today.
2. Canonization of people – The preceding was especially effective if the originating source were an ancient mythical or legendary figure or its mortal representative associated with contemporary religious canon. Hippocrates has been canonized in Western tradition, especially when applied to the Oath.

3. Gate-keepers of canonical knowledge – This type of canonization is relevant today, for these are mortals considered to have special knowledge, insight or prescience that qualify them, according to the political hierarchy, to oversee, maintain and, when necessary, enforce or impose disciplinary guidance. (For an example, see the reference above to Dr. Semmelweis and Prof. Virchow regarding puerperal fever.) As politically centralized government is unavoidably incompetent,[27] its capabilities are confined to selecting from existing knowledge that which is considered favorable from government perspective rather than the citizenry's interest. In doing this, government in effect changes its favored opinion from assertion to fact, *i.e.*, that opinion is canonized. Its factual status will be accepted by those who share the government's perspective. Others may disagree, but they will be unable to challenge it. By this means government agencies have a convenient way to justify on call any particular course of action. In authoritarian governance the knowledge that is canonized will be in those areas considered useful to the political class to gain or retain power. Canonization of knowledge is, in the hands of the gate-keepers, a form of propaganda.

4. Canonization can generate its own popular following, for it can be considered an honor and a privilege to identify with a canon. It is its own elite class because it is exclusionary. Furthermore, to identify with a canon is to assume that bond will not be broken, and such stability is desirable, both socially and economically.

5. Finally, canonization inhibits alternative knowledge and ideas. Governmental canonization not only politicizes and exaggerates the significance of a small portion of available knowledge that it deems useful. It also invalidates the vast store of relevant knowledge that, had it been left alone in medical hands, might have contributed to optimal decision-making.

Canonization is not a feature of just authoritarian societies. The reach of a canon can be broad. In John Donne's poem, *The Canonization*, the poetic lover anticipates generational memory of his efforts in love. Saints, heroes, and other prominent people have been canonized because of the good things they did. Collections of good laws and principles can be designated as canons. Even the political face of a nation can be altered upon an agreement about political canon.[28] So is canonization relevant here?

Canonization can proceed spontaneously if the object is deemed good. Laws agreed to by the people that are useful can be changed when appropriate to keep them "good." Joan of Arc does not need a sociological identifier for us to judge her goodness, although truthful historical documentation is required. Something very good and useful will canonize itself. The issue, therefore, is *purposeful* canonization, which opens the door to canonization of bad ideas and false claims, and *political* canonization, which can propagate those ideas and claims on a vast scale for political purposes and which is the focus of this excursus.

---

[27] For discussion of the inescapable incompetence in government, see excursus 15.

[28] Stuurman, S., *The Canon of the History of Political Thought: It's Critique and a Proposed Alternative*, in *History and Theory*, 39:147-166, 2000.

Political canonization is used to induce sameness into society, the totalitarian's intention as identified by Hannah Arendt.[29] It is not a new idea.[30] It authoritatively limits options on human behavior. It willfully changes opinion into fact, for its argument has been settled by denying legitimacy to alternative arguments, and it acts as an unwritten law unto itself. To willfully promote a canonical issue can be used to exert control over the behavior of others. It also demotes alternative opinions to a lesser status by marginalization or excommunication. By representing its opinion as fact it can inhibit alternative thinking among those who disagree with the canonic issue because its now factual facade can be called upon to justify enforcement, standardization, xenophobia and conscription.

Another consequence of the canonization is its exclusivity. In addition to the misuse of a profession that had a healthy beginning, canonization of medical policies by subsequent authoritarian/totalitarian regimes in the four ancient civilizations inhibited expressions of ingenuity that might have arisen in the unprivileged population. Medical practitioners initially appeared in the common citizenry. One might expect expressions of ingenuity to emerge periodically from the same unprivileged class and therefore a new version of medical profession could periodically reemerge from their ranks. But with a canonized medical presence already in place the possibility that a medical affiliation of several self-styled practitioners might proliferate as a separate, competitive or alternative professional group would be remote.

Lastly, purposeful canonic knowledge is trickle-down knowledge that is determined at higher levels of society (inherently the locus of incompetence) to be appropriate for those in lower levels. This is completely at odds with the Isagorial Theory of Human Progress proposed in *The Natural State of Medical Practice*, in which the source of progress is the collegial association of autonomous individuals with special knowledge in the general population sharing a common interest and having a goal of self-betterment.[31] These individuals, in medicine, would be the practitioners who actually see their patients and have assumed the responsibility for their care. It is these practitioners that produced our Auenbruggers, Laennecs, Pares, Wunderlichs, Listers, and Semmelweises. Those at the top of the social order, the canonizers, are removed from the theater of action and therefore less capable of formulating practical ideas. As an example, by relegating ninety percent of their peasant population to agriculture, Chinese dynastic monarchs disenfranchised the source of most of their kingdoms' ingenuity. Some day someone should try to quantitate this dishonorable and appalling phenomenon.

As human progress is the consequence of a plethora of ideas rather than channeled thinking, purposeful canonization is logically unhealthy. In effect, the underlying political purpose of canonization is to control the thinking of others to the point of sameness, the consequence in medicine being a brake on medical progress. By applying government regulations and guidelines to methods and procedures derived from medical studies, government bypasses that most obvious first step of control, direct command. Instead, and more subtly, it is now government-selected opinion that is canonized, *i.e.*, treated as a fact, and adherence is expected. In medical hands and in medical associations it would not be treated so. It would instead be updated and corrected and we would then find some regulations and guidelines useful, some not, but they would

---

[29] Arendt, H., *The Origins of Totalitarianism,* Cleveland, 1964, p. 438 (paperback).
[30] Theilmann, J. M., *Political Canonization and Political Symbolism in Medieval England*, in J. Brit. Studies, 29:241-266, 1990.
[31] See Excursus 12 for more on the Isagorial Theory of Human Progress.

not be canonized and they would be applied as indicated rather than as directed. When, however, specific medical practice issues are targeted as meriting bureaucratic management, canonization using the definition "only acceptable format" as applied or implied by government regulation is intrusion from outside the profession, one in which inapt methods and procedures become enforceable.

Corporatism:

How can government opinion be efficiently canonized without invoking the medical profession? It does this by inserting itself indirectly into medical practice. It makes itself indispensable by dispensing privileges to selected special interests in return for their allegiance, and it makes them complicit in the consequences. And, like the pharaohs, it can enlist physicians as its mouthpiece. Like the Chinese dynasties, it can insinuate its own ethical, philosophical and economic goals into physician education and research, and like all totalitarian states it can make deals with special interests in which their autonomy is ceded for a guarantee of state support, ultimately financial. The latter mechanism, corporatism, has become more obvious in the age of democratic governance; Hammurabi didn't have to bargain, whereas Hitler, Mussolini and Putin did.

> CORPORATISM: "a system of interest intermediation linking producer interests and the state, in which explicitly recognized interest organizations are incorporated into the policy-making process …" (Oxford Concise Dictionary).

Corporatism in American medicine has been evolving over the last sixty years. Initiation of Medicare with its contributions required by law as medical insurance for the over-65 by the federal government in 1965 began the process. Next came the Health Maintenance Organizations in 1973 in which government acted as a liaison between patients and healthcare providers. Then followed incremental attempts to control costs of medical care, managed care companies, and bundling of services, and 2010 saw, in the Affordable Care Act, far greater integration of relevant businesses into government schemes, a major event in the corporatism process through which government is now close to controlling all medical care throughout the nation.[32] Like the medical guilds in monarchical domains under Hindu medical canon, the individual practitioner is being regulated into conformity by a profession-government complex, aided by certain medical journals (examples of the aforementioned "lease-holders of medicine").[33, 34]

---

[32] The hazards of *The Patient Protection and Affordable Health Care Act* were promptly recognized and articulated by Clete DiGiovanni, MD, and Robert Moffit, PhD, in *How Obamacare Empowers the Medicare Bureaucracy: What Seniors and Their Doctors Should Know*, in WebMemo of *The Heritage Foundation*, No. 2989, August 24, 2010.

[33] "Corporatism" is mentioned many times in volume 3 of *The Natural State of Medical Practice*, but its use in that volume refers to early urbanization and heterarchical governance in primitive societies with no prior experience with government as such. Thus, emerging commercial, agricultural and service units work together to advance their individual interests in a mutually beneficial way. To the extent that there is a central organizational coordination interacting with peripheral interests, this archaic organization might be considered a form of "primitive corporatism" in that coordination rather than control is its raison d'etre.

[34] At the end of this excursus is appended the contents of the medical journal *Lancet* from early July, 1962, and early July, 2022. In the former there **22** articles and letters to the editor that

Corporatism's medical canon, effected or affected by government, need not be technical. Examples include the following: (1) The canon that there are social goals in medical care that justify preferential treatment of patients, thus superseding other aspects of medical care. In the European Dark Ages it was common in religious circles to consider treatment of the soul more important than treatment of the disease. In the Far East a 6th C Confucian physician, Sun Szu Miao, stated "a superior doctor takes care of the state, a mediocre doctor takes care of the person, an inferior doctor takes care of the disease." Corporatism commonly has special interests promoting social goals of government that may favor particular segments of a population. Except for medical triage in disasters where emergency care is preferentially given to the more seriously affected individuals, this is folly, for each person is unique physically, psychologically, medically and potentially, and is to be treated as such. (2) The canon that computerization (*e.g.*, the electronic health record) is the answer for increasing the quality and efficiency of the physician's work. Time and effort is required in fulfilling standardized procedures, of which the medical record is an example; time spent detracts from care of those in need. It also detracts from time necessary to obtain an adequate medical history and physical examination. Its intrusion is also a threat to individualized care when it is used to ensure and document the physician's adherence to guidelines or other ordained standardized approach to patients. (3) The canon that government money is taxpayer money, thereby justifying government regulation of its use by corporate entities. This can affect all aspects of healthcare and is incompatible with the Hippocratic Oath. Only the physician can determine what is medically best for the individual patient, not government committees. Medical practice guided by the Oath and its protection of the physician-patient relation, not a committee of government or special interests, has always been desired and expected by Americans. (4) The Hammurabi approach to medicine ("value-based care") is being copied, *i.e.*, reimbursement is related to outcome, the canon being the better doctors can be identified by their better outcomes. The problem here is ignorance of the variability of humans, of disease, and of humans with disease. This means regulations have the effect of penalizing physicians managing sicker patients and promoting the work of those who would care for those less sick. It follows that the sicker patients are also disadvantaged by value-based care. (5) The canon that there is a best way to manage a disease. Standardized care, while it makes reimbursement and litigation easier, ignores reality in that what may statistically be a favored treatment is absolutely invalidated by two considerations: the weakness inherent in any statistical proof and the variability within the human species. Only the physician can decide the favored treatment for the individual patient.

The preceding can be a disincentive to become a physician if an already rigorous medical education is required to academically integrate sociological concepts unrelated to medical care of the patient. For example, it has been proposed that the modern physician should have a sufficiently comprehensive training in alternative health practices such as holistic, Traditional Chinese Medicine, homeopathy, Ayurveda, and Aromatherapy as well as the standard scientific allopathic medicine. This, plus economic pressures to which corporate interests are particularly sensitive, increases the utilization of those less trained. Ancient Greek physicians had slave assistants who, after hours,

---

specifically involved clinical care; in the latter there was **1**. For the *New England Journal of Medicine* from the same dates the difference is less stark but limited to "articles:" 5 from the 1962 date and **2** from the 2022 date, and one of the latter reported the first genetically modified porcine-to-human cardiac transplantation.

were permitted to provide medical care which they learned by observation to other slaves, if they so wished, in return for reimbursement. Bureaucratic decisions based on economic reasons that promote expansion of patient responsibility to include those with inferior training is another example of bureaucratic incompetence. The public should be aware of the slave physician analogy and its personal relevance the next time they have an appointment to see a Physician Assistant or Nurse Practitioner.[35]

Incompetence, or the consequence of privilege:

A major, but previously understated, problem with government intrusion involves the unprivileged citizenry, the major source of society's competence. Increasing size of government increases the scope of those who are privileged, thus mimicking the persons in the train of dukes, princes, monarchs, and tyrants of dynasties and empires throughout history. This problem is not what government does, which is often bad enough. It is, instead, an unintended consequence. The inherent incompetence of centralized political power, discussed in Excursus 15, increases with its increase in power. With government's focus on regulatory canon, it prevents alternative ideas from being considered. But ingenuity as a national resource is distributed evenly throughout society, and if government regulation and economic policy guide people where it has decided they should go and trains people the way it has decided they should be trained, those people lose their unprivileged status. This might seem to be a big advance, for the unprivileged population shrinks. How can this be viewed otherwise?

In America there should be no inherently privileged population; except that we are privileged to be American, we are all born unprivileged. Protected by the Constitution and the Bill of Rights, every citizen is then free to develop as he or she sees fit. In contrast to preceding civilizations where the unprivileged were in the great majority and any opportunity for self-betterment was thwarted by the privileged, Western civilization constrained somewhat the ambitions of the privileged. This was best achieved, ultimately, in America, where, with no constitutionally inherent privileged class, there was a flood of invention and discovery released around the nation by the general population.

But in the past century this has changed. Many of the population have acquired privileged status by accepting government employment and benevolence and are voluntarily surrendering to government their opportunities for self-betterment, the workshop of human ingenuity. As a result, that portion of our unprivileged society, which is the source of invention and discovery, has greatly decreased as it has increasingly achieved privileged status. As for employment, including the military, fifteen percent of the American labor force is in government employ. We need and want government employees, including those in medicine. They are valuable, but there are limits. Many millions more enjoy government largess and in a sense are government recruits. The larger the total number of the privileged becomes, the more difficult it is to resist socialization of all essential services. Our genie of ingenuity and competence is once again being pushed back into its bottle and the progeny of the newly privileged will bear the sorry consequences.

---

[35] I have worked with many excellent Physician Assistants and Nurse Practitioners. No matter how "nice" they are, the issue is their autonomy and level of supervision. California now (2022) has a law permitting nurse practitioners to perform a first trimester abortion technique without supervision by a physician.

Destabilization:

A serious mechanism for loss of progress distinct from canonization is destabilization of society. Feuds and wars waged by the privileged classes limit the ability of unprivileged individuals to engage in self-betterment and to organize in specializations to the benefit of society as a whole because all of society is focused on survival and the unprivileged have no choice but to march where told. In place of many individual conflicts that can be decided by legislation, the political hierarchy of authoritarianism ignores the natural desire for independence of the individual and can come into conflict with large segments of society and with other authoritarian societies. The resulting national political and civil turmoil disrupts efforts of individuals in society to improve their status or achieve long-term goals, instead enlisting them into that deemed essential for national survival, a necessarily immediate goal. In recent history military decisions concerning initiating a war have usually fallen into the hands of one person. Not only does this person epitomize the pinnacle of the locus of incompetence inherent in authoritarian governance, but negotiations that naturally involve strategic thinking will involve a similar incompetent who leads the opposition. Add to this war initiated by two incompetents the costs of preparation, reparation and reconstruction. The damage to society is unfathomable above and beyond physical devastation. Destabilization is not an immediate problem in American medicine because America's strength among world powers provides stability for all democratic nations. Should that deterrence be weakened to where America becomes just another country, or should centralization of political power continue, conflict will be inevitable and broad, as will its negative consequences on medical progress and practice in America and everywhere else. These comments are not meant to diminish the responsibility of citizens of a democracy to come to its defense.[36]

Summary statement

This excursus has briefly summarized the history of medical practice, which has been, up until the 18th C, a history of misadventure followed by tragedy. From this history I have drawn several conclusions that may be relevant to modern medicine. Since the 18th C we have seen a remarkable blossoming of medical progress. But if intrusion by third parties, especially government and its supportive network, continues as it has, history suggests our profession is on the path to mediocrity equivalent to ancient Ayurveda or Traditional Chinese Medicine. That history is also a warning to other professions and ultimately to the nation. We are actively and passively coming under the aegis of a voracious political class. Canonization, corporatism, and incompetence are doing their malicious work. Many of us are already functioning, often unwittingly and in varying degrees, as its mouthpiece. As a consequence, alternative and complementary medicine are increasingly popular, medical research and medical training are increasingly funded,

---

[36] There have been academic studies that revolve around the Democratic Peace Theory, a theory based on the contention that democracies do not war on other democracies, surely a "good," and while democracy is not the equivalent of freedom it is at the least a step away from authoritarian governance. There are critics of that theory, both theoretical and factual, but at present the dominant opinion is that the Democratic Peace Theory is reasonably supported by evidence. See: Rummel, R., *Never Again: Ending War, Democide, & Famine through Democratic Freedom*, Llumina Press, Coral Springs (FL), 2005, and Gat, A., *War in Human Civilization*, New York, 2006.

and thereby guided, by governmental policy or favorites, and the quality of our work in the office is deteriorating, as suggested by public dissatisfaction and by general medical journals that seem to have gained in political stature what they have lost in clinical relevance (see appendix to this excursus).

Trust in the goodwill of centralized government into the foreseeable future seems to be established despite centuries of evidence that for the common man and woman this is not a good idea. It will be a shame to have reversed what we have recently accomplished. The most striking objective evidence of progress in medicine is increasing life expectancy of the general population:

Mean Stature in Feet and Median Life Span in Years of Humans in Prehistory and History[37]

	Mean Stature (ft.)		Median Life Expectancy (yrs.)	
	M	F	M	F
Paleolithic	5.81	5.47	35.4	30.0
Mesolithic	5.66	5.24	33.5	31.3
Early Neolithic	5.57	5.10	33.6	29.8
Late Neolithic	5.29	5.06	33.1	29.2
Bronze/Iron Ages	5.46	5.06	37.2	31.1
Hellenistic	5.64	5.13	41.9	38.0
Medieval	5.56	5.15	37.7	31.1
Baroque	5.65	5.18	33.9	28.5
19th C	5.58	5.17	40.0	38.4
Late 20th C (USA)	5.72	5.36	**71.0**	**78.5**

The increase in life expectancy was first detected in the Western Europe in the 19th C, Eastern Europe in the 20th C, and now is found in many populations around the world It was not due to the genius of a few great men. It was not built on the shoulders of our ancestors. It certainly was not directed by political leadership or government; in fact, it was just the opposite. No government can ever claim it has contributed to progress, period. And it was not due to necessity, for that necessity has always been with us. It also was not due to an increasingly intelligent and benevolent humankind. We are no kinder or wiser than our distant ancestors. It has been due to one thing, and one thing only, and that is a freeing of the common man and woman from their anonymous servility that has characterized their social status since the first human societies. It has been their escape from the strong bonds of kinship and stronger bonds of authoritarian governance. It is clear that the increase in life expectancy followed, rather than preceded, the early progress of Western medicine. And this great transformation took place in the West.[38] Of course, improved sanitation, productive agriculture, and less physical risk in tasks of daily living have contributed to our well-being, but the source of their improvements is the same although medicine takes the prize.

[37] This Table is modified from that used by: Wells, S., in *Pandora's Seed: The Unforeseen Cost of Civilization*, New York, 2010, p. 23. Measurements of stature could reflect nutritional status.
[38] Justification for this statement is a separate issue, but the initial argument is found in Excursus 8.

Throughout history, however, centralization of power and placing it in hands of the locus of incompetence has led us into perpetual cul-de-sacs. Much more can be said about the tragic history of the common citizenry on this point, but for present purposes it is sufficient to declare that within our profession **we must (1) protect the *sanctum sanctorum* of the physician-patient relation, (2) prevent those outside of the profession from controlling it, (3) remove it from all political issues by limiting its scope to its core principles, (4) forbid any political collaboration or coercion, whether by government or its proxy, special interests, (5) compete with, but do not join with or proscribe, alternative forms healthcare practices, (6) focus on clinical medicine, (7) vigorously maintain professional standards, and (8) remain true to the Hippocratic Oath.**

With government, alternative medicine, major medical associations, and a politically susceptible and unsuspecting public threatening traditional medical practice, matters do appear grim. Change will be difficult. It also will never be complete. The best that can be done is to reverse such matters as we can, little by little. This will be greatly expedited when private medical practices are shown to be more effective and increasingly requested than alternative practices. Medical schools especially must adapt. Increase the visibility of the praiseworthy efforts of our professionals and disparage the perilous efforts of the authoritarians. This is not the time to be modest. The democracy between physicians and patients must be restored. We can return to modesty when we have repaired the perimeters of our profession and reunited the physician-patient relation. Meanwhile we must spread the word of just what will happen if matters continue as they are, and, to repeat the words of Richard Hurrell Froude:

"Open your eyes to the fearful change which has been so noiselessly affected; and acknowledge BY STANDING STILL YOU BECOME A PARTY TO REVOLUTION." (sic)

Richard Hurrell Froude (1803-1836)[39]

---

[39] Hurrell Froude was the elder brother of the famous English historian, James Anthony Froude. A cleric, Hurrell's statement is to be found in *Remarks on State interference in Matters Spiritual*, in *Remains of the Late Reverend Richard Hurrell Froude, M. A.*, vol. I of Part 2, Derby, 1839, p. 196. Although pertaining to "matters spiritual," Froude adds the comment, based on the principles of Hooker, that it "goes to any kind of State interference at all." Froude, part of the early 19th C Oxford Movement in England, was arguing a principle of 16th C Calvinism.

Appendix:

For comparison of medical journals of the recent past and present, here are listed the contents of articles in two issues of two prominent medical journals. The first issue was published the week I began my internship in 1962, the second issue sixty years later:

LANCET, first issue of July 1962
Articles
The Negative Symptoms of Basal Gangliar Disease (survey of 130 postencephalitic cases)
Iron Absorption in Pancreatic Disease
Steroid Therapy in Heart-block Following Myocardial Infarction
Blood Lavage in Acute Barbiturate Poisoning (ten years experience)
Gritti-Stokes Amputation for Atherosclerotic Gangrene
Heritable Variation in the Length of the Y Chromosome
Absence of the Y Chromosome (X0 Sex-Chromosome Constitution) in a Human Intersex
        with an Extra-Abdominal Testis
The Minicoil Artificial Kidney
Haematological Factors as Related to the Sex Difference in Coronary-Artery Disease
Apparatus for Nursing Infants Upright
                   (10 articles, average number of authors per article: 2)
Letters to the editor
Pulmonary-embolic Disease
Thalidomide-damaged Babies
Placental Monoamine-oxidase activity and toxaemia of pregnancy
Threadworms
Practice in Saskatchewan
RIpH
The Aged Motorist
Information on Toxicity
Neuropsychologists in Medical Schools
Efficiency of Cardiac Massage
Sodium-retainin Steroids in Non-edematous Patients
Trends in Mental-Hospital Population and their effect on Planning
Citrullinuria in cases of cystinuria
HP
Films on Mental-health Subjects
Surgery of Road Accidents
Irritant Properties of Wescodyne
Snuff
Reactions with Phenindione
The Real Problem of Migraine
Testicular Changes in Infant of Diabetic Mother
Activities of the X Chromosome
Satellites of Acrocentric Chromosomes
Aetiology of Choriocarcinoma
Cervical Spondylosis: A Requesdt for Pathological Material

LANCET, first issue of July, 2022
Articles
Live Expectancy by County, Race and Ethnicity in the USA, 2000-19: A Systematic Analysis of Health Disparities
Immobilization of Torus Fractures of the Wrist in Children (FORCE): A Randomised Controlled Equivalence Trial in the UK
Effectiveness of Interventions to improve Drinking Water, Sanitation, and Handwashing with Soap on the Risk of Diarrhoeal Disease in Children in Low-Income and Middle-Income Settings: A Systematic Review and Meta-Analysis
(3 articles, average number of authors per article: 19)
Correspondence
Guidelines for Pregnant Individuals with Monkeypox Virus Exposure
Monkeypox Genomic Surveillance Will Challenge Lessons Learned from SARS-CoV-2
The Monkeypox Outbreak Must Amplify Hidden Voices in the Global Discourse
Shifting Gender Barriers in Immunisation in the COVID-19 Pandemic Response and Beyond

NEJM, first issue of July, 1962
Articles
Evaluation of Tri-Iodothyronine in the Treatment of Acute Alcoholic Intoxication
Idiopathic Hemosiderosis – Relation to idiopathic Hemochromatosis
Chronic Postrheumatic-Fever (Jaccoud's) Arthritis
Arteriovenous Fistula of the Aortic Arch
Hemorrhagic State Due to Surreptitious Ingestion of Bishydroxycoumarin
(5 articles, average number of authors per article: 2)
Correspondence
Mission Accomplished   (re: angina pectoris)
Paging M. Poirot
Infant Wetback
Credit for Research Grant
A Correction
Hamartomata Galore

NEJM, first issue of July, 2022
Articles
Trastuzumab Deruxtecan in Previously Treated HER2-Low Advanced Breast Cancer
Effects of Previous Infection and Vaccination on Symptomatic Omicron Infections
Brief Report: Genetically Modified Porcine-to-Human Cardiac Xenotransplantation
(3 articles, average number of authors per article: 12 et al.)
Correspondence
Neutralization Escape by SARS-CoV-2 Omicron Subvariants BA.2.12.1, BA.4, and BA.5
SARS-CoV-2 Infection in Patients with a History of VITT
Nonoperative or Surgical Treatment of Acute Achilles' Tendon Rupture
The Increasing Incidence of Early-Onset Colorectal Cancer
Prone Positioning of Intubated Patients with an Elevated BMI

EXCURSUS 18[1]

We are all descendants of both slaves and enslavers. In its briefest terms, this excursus acknowledges enslavement as a common component of all past civilizations. At the same time, natural law makes clear to every person that enslavement is immoral. The explanation for this seeming paradox is that natural law has been overruled by positive (man-made) laws and actions imposed by authoritarian dictate. The Ten Commandments (the Decalogue) are a formal exposition of natural law expressed in Judeo-Christian scripture, and they affirmed the abnegation of slavery to the West. Yet enslavement persisted. But the Reformation then declared the equal status of all persons before God, following which secular leadership and citizens began to be viewed as equals and equally subject to natural law. As legislatures became more representative of their citizens, natural law was increasingly incorporated into secular laws defending natural rights. Remarkably, just as it took two-and-a-half centuries after the onset of the Reformation for modern medical progress to appear, the same period was required for abolitionism to be initiated on a national scale. Morality and ingenuity of the common citizenry were unleashed simultaneously. Such is the power of associations of a free people when endowed with natural rights and guided by natural law instead of authoritarian governance run by a privileged political class. The abolition of slavery, like medical progress, can thus be explained by the *Isagorial Theory of Human Progress*, which now seems to encompass the political as well as apolitical betterment of mankind.[2] Although the preceding is a Western drama unique in the history of civilizations, the Judeo-Christian Decalogue, as a formal statement of natural law, is the birthright of all humanity.

THE REFORMATION, ENSLAVEMENT, AND THE ISAGORIAL THEORY OF HUMAN PROGRESS

Introduction

It is frequently pointed out that enslavement is as old and widespread as mankind.[3] There is no one who is not the descendant of many slaves. Most of those slaves would have been from conquered populations. And it is likely that most of those ancestors were women, for in many instances it was the female who was enslaved. It is for this reason that Professor Orlando Patterson proposed that the first true appreciation of, and voice for, individual liberty was that of women, for they knew and lived the horrors

---

[1] Volume and page number of otherwise unreferenced statements in this monograph refer to the version of the three volumes of *The Natural State of Medical Practice* as published by Liberty Hill Press in 2019:
Vol. 1 – *The Natural State of Medical Practice: An Isagorial Theory of Human Progress*
Vol. 2 – *The Natural State of Medical Practice: Hippocratic Evidence*
Vol. 3 - *The Natural State of Medical Practice: Escape from Egalitarianism*
[2] Definition of *Isagorial Theory of Human Progress*: A theory ascribing all apolitical advances for the betterment of mankind to autonomous associations pursuing self-betterment in which each member has equal opportunity to speak freely and share ideas about the group's common interest without fear of retribution. Axiomatically it excludes "betterments" that have been stolen, copied, derived by exploitation, or used for subjugation of others. (See Excursus 12, Validation of the Isagorial Theory of Human Progress.)
[3] Hunt, P., *Slavery*, in *The Cambridge World History*, volume 4:76-100.

of slavery. The men had been spared that injustice; whether in battle or as prisoners afterward, they were all killed.[4]

The converse of the above is also true. There is no one who is not the descendant of many enslavers. Indeed, the very fact that each of us, the living, exist is in all likelihood testimony to the success of some of our ancestors in enslaving some of their contemporaries, thus enabling a few of those ancestors to survive and procreate. The prehistory and history of mankind is so teeming with threats to survival, and the ability of our species to survive amidst them has been so pitiful (as demonstrated in Excursus 9, "After Eden," and in volume 3 of *The Natural State of Medical Practice,* p. 211*ff*), that it could be argued that humans as a species might have become extinct without the enforced subjugation of others at critical periods.[5]

It has always been easy enough to find examples of enslavers among Western Christian, Orthodox Christian, Islamic, Hindu, Buddhist, Confucian, Zoroastrian, pre-Columbian polytheistic civilizations, ancient Egyptian polytheism, Tengrism (which includes shamanism and animism), and Shinto religious practices. As enslavement has been a global practice, therefore, the question is not the morality of those who practiced it, for that would include ancestors of all of us, and it is we in the West who formally came to know the answer: it was immoral. The real question is, who formally, *i.e.,* through legislation, effectively outlawed slavery based on moral grounds rather than merely expedient ones.

Source of moral argument

There were many early opinions critical of enslavement, and they are frequent enough to conclude that there is in the consciences of mankind a natural antipathy to enslavement, an awareness by every individual that it is a bad thing to do. Many prominent Greeks and Romans expressed humane concerns depending on the type of enslavement. But the institution of slavery was not confronted as a universal nemesis, although Zeno, the stoic philosopher, (*ca.* 300 BC) considered it "despicable," and the Mauryan Buddhist king Ashoka (3rd C BC) stopped the trading of slaves in the Indian subcontinent. Indeed, there are expressions by individuals in the ancient history of every civilization in every age and region desiring an end to or moderation of slavery. It is a reasonable conclusion that the moral argument against enslavement is found in the conscience of every person, which is natural law.

Natural law contains the same message about right and wrong that is found in the Ten Commandments (herein the Decalogue), the distinction being that the Decalogue

---

[4] Patterson, O., *Freedom in the Making of Western Culture*, New York, 1991, Part II, *The Greek Construction of Freedom.*

[5] This perhaps odd suggestion may be relevant to the absence of an abolitionist stance against slavery in the Bible, especially regarding the Decalogue, the Covenant Code, and relevant commentary. The immediate and complete cessation of any form of slavery might have been considered lethal by inhabitants of relevant societies. A society's abolition of slavery in a world where slavery was everywhere established might have led to that society's disappearance. An analogy might be today's Quaker population in America. As a profoundly pacifist society its members are conscientious objectors to participation in warfare, but should America with its protective forces lose its autonomy to an authoritarian State, Quakerism would be one of the earliest of sectarian groups to be regulated into anonymity.

is not subliminal. It is written in stone, so to speak. Evidence of the immorality of slavery is found in the 1st and 8th Commandments (the latter being one of the "ethical" Commandments and states, "you do not take from others" (οὐ κλέψεις). The Decalogue was directed at every Hebrew and forbade the individual from taking something from someone else (without their permission). This could be property, livelihood, reputation or freedom (as a natural right) itself. We need look no further for a moral denouncement of slavery as evil. [6]

It is fair to state, therefore, that judgment on slavery as good vs. bad or right vs. wrong or moral vs. immoral is not an arbitrary thing. It is immoral and everyone knows it and has always known it. To claim not to know it is a guilty verdict on the society to which one belongs. And in the past that judgment can be applied to every society and every civilization. This was to end.

Setting the stage

Despite natural law and despite the Decalogue, enslavement in various forms continued everywhere and motives were, in general, related to the status of citizen vs. noncitizen as implemented or facilitated by positive (man-made) laws, whether at a domain or a tribal level. Although there is considerable academic controversy, the Decalogue has been dated to the 13th C BC following the exodus of the Hebrews from Egypt under Moses. But there was limited social response to this Commandment that would abolish slavery, in part because of disruptions and captivities of Hebrew tribes themselves.

Nevertheless, the Jewish population of the Roman Empire grew to be several millions and the Decalogue remained prominent in Jewish writing for all to see, including the works of Philo (20 BC-50 AD) and Josephus (37-100 AD). Most important, via the Pentateuch it was prominently transmitted to Christianity.

It was for the Judeo-Christian religion to first oppose enslavement as an institution. The Essenes, a Jewish sect *ca.* 100 BC, did formally forbid its practice and opposed it on moral grounds. The Essene population was not large, but it was an integral part of the Jewish community, and Prof. Timothy Lim considers this to have been a unique principled stand.[7] St. Paul (1st C AD) then stated (Luke 6.31) "And as ye would that men should do to you, do ye also to them likewise."[8] As Martin Luther would later interpret it: "Therefore, I cannot strip another of his possessions, no matter how clear a right I have, so long as I am unwilling myself to be stripped of my goods. Rather, just as I would that another, in such circumstances, should relinquish his right in my favor, even so should I relinquish my rights."[9]

---

[6] Continuing with the proposal of the previous footnote, this might explain some biblical allusions to slavery that advise kindness to the enslaved rather than outright abolition of slavery in early civilization, for its presence was universal and viewed by many as necessary. To have it abolished might have been considered suicidal by contemporary reasoning. It would take a civilization based on the Decalogue to overcome this presumed obligatory requisite for survival.

[7] Lim, T., *The Earliest Commentary on the Prophecy of Habakkuk,* Oxford, 2021.

[8] This is a restatement of the "Golden Rule" which, as discussed in Excursus 6, can also be equated to natural law and to the Decalogue.

[9] Excerpted from Luther's *Temporal Authority: To What Extent It Should Be Obeyed.* (1523)

Gregory of Nyssa, a 4th C Bishop and Church Father from the center of modern Turkey, also considered it as an affront to God, of Whom every person was a creation. He traced his opinions on slavery to the earlier teachings of Origen of Alexandria (185-253 AD), a Church Father who agreed with freeing of the enslaved in the seventh year as expressed in the Pentateuch, and in his *De Principiis*, Book 3, concluded that mankind possessed free will to deal with its responsibilities and therefore needed to be free to do so.

But in the post-Roman West dialogue regarding both the Decalogue and slavery through the Dark Ages and Medieval Period was limited because most of the population were already serfs. During those centuries, the widespread Christian kinship under the aegis of the Roman Catholic Church had little to say either *pro* or *con* slavery.[10] This is explained in part by the myriad of small communities throughout post-Roman Europe inhabited primarily by poor peasants with pre-assigned obligations within a self-sustaining feudal system that would have provided no home for imported slaves.

Later there was a Germanic legal code, *Sachsen Spiegel* (*ca.* 1220), that expressed the same opinion as the Church, that humans were "a likeness of God," but, as discussed by Prof. Hans Frambach, it specifically condemned "the total power of one man over another." Aspects of this law code, which reflected ancient Saxon tradition and law of a free people, had parallels to English common law. A few institutions and city-states also prohibited or limited serfdom and sometimes slavery. Natural law was peeping through the curtain. But overall there was limited experience in Europe with overt slavery even though during the Crusades extensive slavery was encountered by Christian armies, with varying degrees of accommodation in the Near East.

But as the second millennium proceeded, two important trends were under way. In one it was increasingly recognized in the West that, with the Decalogue gaining prominence and its equivalence with natural law clearly identified by Thomas Aquinas (1225-1274), the importance of personal responsibility rather than tribal dictate in following its Commandments was being recognized. In the other, especially in the 14th and 15th centuries, there was a developing European economy based on a growing population and mercantilism, and trade and colonization could particularly benefit from slavery. Slavery as an institution was now visible and relevant to more and more of the general population. There were occasional attempts to stop participation in local or regional enslavements, but with monarchical powers favoring trade practices that benefited from the labors of enslaved populations, a sustained policy forbidding slavery did not emerge.

Meanwhile, questioning of the authority of the Church proceeded apace. The Hussites, the Lollards, and the humanism of the Renaissance (the "anticlerical" writings of Erasmus preceded Martin Luther) were disruptions, physical and intellectual, that occupied the Church hierarchy. But slavery remained an unimportant issue. Erasmus (1466-1536) wrote a *paraphrasis* in 1519 of St. Paul's letter concerning Onesimus, a runaway slave who stole items from his master but became Paul's "equal" upon his baptism, but there is no comment by Erasmus on slavery *per se* in the text where Paul mediates the return of Onesimus to his master.

---

[10] A similar argument would apply to the troubled centuries of the ancient Hebrews, namely the disruptive centuries characterized by wars, captivity, and Roman desolation. The Decalogue was always there, in oral, then written, tradition, but the laws of men, the positive laws of authoritarian regimes, would shield them from its full observance.

It has been suggested by some that the Reformation was inevitable, a natural consequence of earlier anticlerical efforts. On the other hand, Luther's initial call for resolution of his ecclesiastical concerns, had it been answered with some concessions, may have prevented the subsequent schism within the Church and brought about a more acceptable relation between feudal leaders and the Church, thereby strengthening the *status quo*. Perhaps this will be clarified in the future, but the very fact of the Reformation would now alter European society forever, and, for the West, this would include for the first time in history legislation abolishing slavery on moral grounds.

Moral orientation of the Reformation

What is Christian morality? The range of opinion is considerable, and there is variation in its definition depending on religious denomination and on the mores of contemporary society. But there is some academic agreement that in the early Medieval Period (500-1000 AD) it was the Seven Deadly Sins that were prominent in its definition, whereas as the centuries passed the Decalogue gradually became, and remains, dominant.

Three important features are considered relevant here. One is the idea that the Decalogue was specifically directed at the individual, requiring one to personally assess his or her actions as good or bad, whereas the Seven Deadly Sins were straightforward "do nots" emanating from society's religious leadership. There was no equivocation and no searching of the conscience necessary.[11] Second, this change to the Decalogue involved the element of introspection, an appeal to the individual to determine the appropriateness of an action, a source of informed choice; personal choice broadened its scope and identified one's judge as God, not an official. And third, this approach became practical when Bibles became available in the vernacular, for now the average person could have direct access to knowledge of process rather than being prescribed a "rule of conduct."[12]

Thus, the Decalogue, which had been considered by Thomas Aquinas to be the equivalent of natural law and an appropriate statement on Christian morality, became increasingly prominent. This was clearly evident in the writings of Martin Luther. Calvin also expressed it with regularity and even increased its prominence by promoting musical versions (he viewed music as an effective vehicle for spreading the Word). And as the Reformation spread throughout northern Europe Queen Elizabeth in 1560 ordered that the Ten Commandments be prominently posted in every church in England. This was reaffirmed by James I, and then Charles II, during the Restoration and despite a turn from Calvinist practices, ordered that they be posted in every church that he had ordered rebuilt by Christopher Wren following the great fire of London in 1666. Their location was specified so as to be obvious to everyone, and repetitions were part of liturgy.[13] Prominent also during Elizabeth's reign and contemporary Europe was iconoclasm, as destruction of

---

[11] Briefly, they are: pride, greed, lust, envy, gluttony (drunkenness), wrath and sloth.

[12] *The Ten Commandments in Medieval and Early Modern Culture*, Leiden 2017, Y. Desplenter, J. Pieters, W. Melion, eds., see Introductory chapter.

[13] These interesting observations were reported by Drew Keane in his article, *Commandment Boards and Catechesis*, in *The North American Anglican*. It has also been pointed out that humanist ideas were afloat during the Renaissance, and the dominance of the Church was being questioned by intellectuals of the 15th C. Henry VIII was attracted to this way of thinking, and it was this, rather than Reformation thinking, that led to his anticlerical reign.

statues, paintings and other popular manifestations of saints and other venerable items was considered justified based on the Second Commandment, either as examples of idols or as a source of temptation.

It can be concluded that the Decalogue, at least with the onset of the Reformation, was now considered the formal expression of and vessel for Christian morality.[14] Natural law was no longer to be easily ignored.

The Reformation and slavery

For background, the consequences of the release of human ingenuity following the onset of the Reformation are subjects of Excursus 8 which traced the concepts of natural rights and equality of all people in determining their own governance from the equality of all persons before God. Thus, religious leaders and their congregants were equals within the Church. It was the Reformation that would lead some to conclude the same applied to the secular world; the leader must obey the same higher authority as the citizen and could be ousted if he did not. What ultimately followed was legislative protection of religious rights and then natural rights of the individual, thereby freeing the great majority of the population to pursue self-betterment rather than the betterment of their betters. Evidence of ingenuity of individuals and the formation of collegial associations for providing specialized crafts and services appeared. As discussed in *The Natural State of Medical Practice* (vol. 1), these associations were distinct from the protective guilds of medieval cities. In particular, medical practices and associations began to appear, displacing in the public mind the bogus medicine and bogus physicians of Late Medieval universities. The field of medicine began to evolve a natural state of medical practice and the 18th C saw the early flourishing of ingenuity in medical care that would peak in the 20th C. To this we can attribute medical progress, our longevity, and modern conveniences and prosperity. Thus, I propose the timeline of the freedoms of the West to extend from the Mosaic Decalogue to the present day, justifying the concept of a Judeo-Christian Civilization rather than a Western one (see Excursus 16).

This excursus argues that the same sequence applies to slavery, concluding that the moral eradication of slavery is solely a consequence of the Judeo-Christian civilization and the morality of the Decalogue. The democratic trends of the ancient Greeks were irrelevant in furthering abolition of slavery because their philosophical renderings regarding slavery were of no practical value. Unmistakably, the issue has always been moral rather than political, but political machinations have prevented its proper recognition. No other civilization or culture on earth has taken such a principled stand on slavery's abolition.

Martin Luther in the 16th C did not dwell on the institution of slavery, perhaps in part because he considered all mankind as slaves (of the Devil) until that moment that faith led to salvation. His colleague, Philip Melanchthon (1497-1560), however, made the position clear: "Also in civil law, as they call it, there are many things that reflect human affections instead of natural laws. For what is more foreign to the law of nature than slavery? ....a good man will fashion civil constitutions according to a just and good

---

[14] The Reformation prompted many Christians to declare the Decalogue as irrelevant to Christianity, for it was considered specifically directed at the Hebrews. It and its attached ritual and social commentary were thought outmoded. In the Reformation it was natural law, therefore, that reigned in its place, even though Luther himself equated the two.

rule, that is, with both divine and natural laws. And whatever is instituted against these laws can be nothing but unjust."[15]

Luther's equality of leader and the led, directed at Church hierarchy, was promptly echoed throughout the reforming churches of northern Europe, profoundly aided by the printing press. Instigatory tracts were published. An early publication was *Vindiciae Contra Tyrannos*, a Huguenot tract of 1578.[16] In *Lex, Rex*, a 1644 book by a Protestant minister in Scotland, Samuel Rutherford, clearly stated in Question 40 that "The prince is but a private man in a contract" and that a king is not a king until he takes an oath and is "accepted by the people." But beyond this, "A man being created according to God's image, he is *res sacra*, a sacred thing, and can no more, by nature's law, be sold and bought, than a religious or sacred thing dedicated to God." The equality of the religious leader and the led was being politically duplicated with the ruler and the ruled. Rules were changing.

Once triggered by Luther because of simony within the Church, much of Europe underwent massive institutional changes, especially in political and economic arenas that would seem to be social venues quite distinct from religion. How could this happen?

With new limitations on the power of the Roman Church in some regions because of the Reformation, local political leadership, usually the traditional elite hierarchy, looked to other institutions to support its continued financing and governance. Parliaments were enlisted to help. Although knowledge of early events of the Reformation on the continent was available in England, it was Henry VIII that removed the label of heresy by introducing aspects of the Reformation into the English system of government. He used Parliament for that purpose, the consequence being that now Parliament would approve monarchical plans rather than Papal concurrence. Parliaments thereby increased their influence.

During this contentious period the Roman Church was not indifferent to natural law and the Decalogue and their implications for freedom. The statement was made at the Council of Trent (1545-1563): "Since then, the Decalogue is a summary of the whole Law, the pastor should give his days and nights to its consideration that he might be able not only to regulate his own life by its precepts, but also to instruct in the law of God the people committed to his care."

There had been a gradual release from much of serfdom in western European populations prior to the Reformation, and it was possible to purchase freedom. Even some cities were able to afford their separation from feudal control. In contrast, eastern Europe serfdom was slower to appear and late to disappear, with aspects of serfdom common into the 18th and 19th centuries. Thus, while serfdom is not the same as slavery, it appears that neither the Reformation nor the Roman Church *per se*, as a religious movement or an institution, can claim to have directly contributed to abolition. Instead, change would come from the message of the Decalogue as implemented by its recipients, the congregants, the general citizenry, rather than institutional leadership.

In 1524 the first dialogue of the *Doctor and Student* appeared in England. Written by a "Protestant" who would ultimately be considered a "reformer," Christopher St. Germain (1460-1540), the work was the first to analyze English common law and natural law, thereby influencing William Blackstone as well as our Founding Fathers. In Dialogue I, chap. 2, he wrote:

---

[15] *Commonplaces: Loci Communes*, 1521, transl. Christian Preus (St. Louis: CPH, 2014), p. 66.

[16] This website, **contratyrannos.com**, derives its name from that work, the author presumed to be Hubert Languet, a "French reformer" but born in Antwerp in 1518.

Doct. The law of reason teacheth, that good is to be loved, and evil is to be fled: also that thou shalt do to another, that thou wouldest another should do unto thee; and that we may do nothing against truth; and that a man must live peacefully with others; that justice is to be done to every man; and also that wrong is not to be done to any man; and that also a trespasser is worthy to be punished; and such other. Of the which follow divers other secondary commandments, the which be as necessary conclusions derived of the first. As of that commandment, that good is to be beloved; it followeth, that a man should love his benefactor: for a benefactor, in that he is a benefactor, includeth in him a reason of goodness, for else he ought not to be called a benefactor; that is to say, a good doer, but an evil doer: and so in that he is a benefactor, he is to be beloved in all times and in all places. And this law also suffereth many things to be done: as that it is lawful to put away force with force; and that it is lawful for every man to defend himself and his goods against an unlawful power. And this law runneth with every man's law [positive law], and also with the law of God [the Decalogue], as to the deeds of man, and must be always kept and observed, and shall always declare what ought to follow upon the general rules of the law of man, and shall restrain them if they be any thing contrary unto it.

The similarity of St. Germain's statement to the Decalogue, natural law, and the Golden Rule is obvious. What the writer considers to be natural law he calls the "law of reason," and by the "law of God" he refers to the Ten Commandments, for the latter were "revealed."

Excursus 16 identifies several writers of the 16th and 17th centuries (*e.g.*, Johannes Althusius, 1563-1638) that recognized the biblical justification of the concept of natural rights. Then John Locke (1632-1704), born to Puritan parents, developed a political philosophy that some consider an important cause of the Enlightenment of the 17th and 18th centuries. His message to us was encapsulated in these words: we have rights to life, liberty, and estate (property). Locke believed in the supremacy of the Bible. In *Two Treatises on Government* (1689), Bk. II, chap. 2, sect. 6., the antislavery sentiment is obvious. He wrote:

The state of nature has a law of nature to govern it, which obliges every one: and reason, which is that law, teaches all mankind, who will but consult it, that being all equal and independent, no one ought to harm another in his life, health, liberty, or possessions: for men being all the workmanship of one omnipotent, and infinitely wise maker; all the servants of one sovereign master, sent into the world by his order, and about his business; they are his property, whose workmanship they are, made to last during his, not one another's pleasure: and being furnished with like faculties, sharing all in one community of nature, there cannot be supposed any such subordination among us, that may authorize us to destroy one another, as if we were made for one another's uses, as the inferior ranks of creatures are for ours. Every one, as he is bound to preserve himself, and not to quit his station willfully, so by the like reason, when his own preservation comes not in competition, ought he, as much as he can, to preserve the rest of mankind, and may not, unless it be to do justice on an offender, take away, or impair the life, or what tends to the preservation of the life, the liberty, health, limb, or goods of another.

It is interesting that neither he nor St. Germain specify the Mosaic Decalogue in their writings. Luther had made clear a reason for this: the Decalogue was from the Old Testament and was revealed specifically to the Hebrews, whereas natural law was the same thing but was engrained in every person. Thus, the Decalogue was a secondary manifestation to a people that needed to have it pointed out. There was reticence to give credit to the Jewish origin of the covenant of the Ten Commandments if its presence was already available to everyone via human reason.

The prominence of natural law was increasing, and what natural law was here to protect was being discussed. Thus, the political focus turned also to natural rights. An early example was the work of Francis Hutcheson (1694-1746), son of a minister, later Professor of Moral Philosophy in Glasgow, who wrote the following in his important work, *An Inquiry into the Original of Our Ideals of Beauty and Virtue* (in Treatise Two, Concerning Moral Good and Evil, sect. 7, VI):

> The Rights call'd perfect, are of such necessity to the publick Good, that the universal Violation of them would make human Life intolerable; and it actually makes those miserable, whose Rights are thus violated. On the contrary, to fulfil these Rights in every Instance, tends to the publick Good either directly, or by promoting the innocent Advantage of a Part. Hence it plainly follows, "That to allow a violent Defence, or Prosecution of such Rights, before Civil Government be constituted, cannot in any particular Case be more detrimental to the Publick, than the Violation of them with Impunity." And as to the general Consequences, the universal Use of Force in a State of Nature, in pursuance of perfect Rights, seems exceedingly advantageous to the Whole by making every one dread any Attempts against the perfect Rights of others.

Concurrently, Montesquieu ((1689-1755) in his *Esprit des Lois* (Bk. 15) noted "Slavery is moreover as contrary to civil law as to natural law." On the other hand, after discussing the variety of enslavement, he concludes: "But whatever be the nature of the slavery, civil law must try to free it from abuses...." Adam Smith (1723-1790) viewed the problem analytically and argued slavery was not economically efficient but unlikely to be stopped because of laziness of the enslavers. So, it may be proposed that in some circles there was a roar of antislavery sentiment but not much bite.

With the increased wealth associated with colonialism and the Reformation, sometimes attributed to the "Protestant work ethic," businesses prospered, and employees were needed to allow supply to match demand. Thus, economic issues have been blamed for the flourishing of the slave trade, but, more recently, a thoughtful explanation for its abolition.[17]

But I propose it is exposure to, experience with, and discussion of slavery occurring among the general citizenry that would ultimately lead to its abolition on *moral* grounds. It has been effectively argued that abolition of the slave trade in the West was possible because of efforts of nonconformist Christians, primarily 18th C Evangelist and Quaker sects in Great Britain and the United States. Quakers and other dissenting groups arose in 17th C England during the mid-century Civil War.[18] Thus, a variety of

---

[17] Williams, E., *Capitalism and Slavery*, Chapel Hill, 2021 (third edition).

[18] Important in leading to abolition were individuals such as James Oglethorpe, Lord Mansfield and Sir John Holt, and a variety of legal suits. But most important were active associations such as Clapham Sect, Quakers, the African Association, the Committee for the Abolition of the Slave Trade, and groups from denominations including Methodists, Baptists, Swedenborgians, and Anglicans. Notably, women and women's groups were, for the first time, activists, although they were ineligible to vote. It has been said that legal abolition in English law was slow in coming, but it should be remembered that few English were eligible to vote because of land requirements. And there were other factors: Manchester's population of 250,000 in 1831 had no Member of Parliament for whom to vote. *A generous estimate is that about one in twenty males could vote at that time.*

associations came to this opinion, and the justification for their stance was founded on their religious morality, the Decalogue and/or natural law.

William Blackstone (1723-1780), an Anglican from a middle-class shop-keeper's family, was profoundly influenced by the Decalogue and its equivalent, natural law. In his magisterial *Commentaries of the Laws of England* (vol. 1, p. 41, 1765) he wrote:

> This law of nature, being co-eval with mankind and dictated by God himself, is of course superior in obligation to any other. It is binding over all the globe, in all countries, and at all times; no human laws are of any validity, if contrary to this; and such of them as are valid derive all their force, and all their authority, mediately or immediately, from this original.

Here Blackstone equates natural law with the Decalogue, the latter as dictated by God and equivalent to St. Germain's Law of God received by revelation. With regard to enslavement, he wrote (ibid., chapter 14, Of Master and Servant): "

> Upon these principles the law of England abhors, and will not endure the existence of, slavery within this nation; so that when an attempt was made to introduce it, by statute 1 Edw. VI. c. 3, which ordained, that all idle vagabonds should be made slaves, and fed upon bread and water, or small drink, and refuse meat; should wear a ring of iron round their necks, arms, or legs; and should be compelled, by beating, chaining, or otherwise, to perform the work assigned them, were it never so vile; the spirit of the nation could not brook this condition, even in the most abandoned rogues; and therefore this statute was repealed in two years afterwards.(d) And now it is laid down,(e) that a slave or negro, the instant he lands in England, becomes a freeman; that is, the law will protect him in the enjoyment of his person, and his property."

Other factors were in play, but I propose it was aspects of Judeo-Christian morality that provided the key justification for abolition as expressed not by Government or Church but in the enthusiasm of the general citizenry when they realized what the problem was and that they were able to do something about it. As Dr. R Anstey has written, "It was mainly religious insight and zeal … which made it possible for anti-slavery feeling to be subsumed in a crusade against the slave trade. [19] It has been argued that economic issues were the explanation for the success of abolition in the late 18th C, but Dr Anstey considered economic explanations to be inadequate. As Abraham Lincoln said, "With public sentiment nothing can fail; without it nothing can succeed. Consequently he who molds public sentiment, goes deeper than he who enacts statutes or pronounces decisions."[20]

The subsequent course of abolitionism is well-described in many publications. But the whole argument revolved around moral issues rather than sectarian or economic ones. People saw that enslavement was the ultimate suppression of natural rights. The immorality of suppression of natural rights is clearly expressed in the Decalogue and in natural law. Whether by law of God, natural law, or, most succinctly, the Golden Rule, the ending of slavery is without question a Western phenomenon based on Judeo-

---

[19] Anstey, R., *The Atlantic Slave Trade and British Abolition, 1760-1810*, Atlantic Highlands (NJ), 1975, (p. 153).
[20] Lincoln-Douglas debates, Ottawa, 1858.

Christianity as first formally expressed in the Mosaic Commandments. Would that it be so recognized globally.

Concluding note: Isagorial Theory and political progress

Why did it, in both medical progress and in abolitionism, take two-and-a-half centuries from the onset of the Reformation for action to follow words? The answer herein is the same for both: it took time for government to get out of the way.[21] Government, while necessary, is never the actual origin of anything good. It can assist in correction of a "bad," and it is proper in its provisions of the necessary, but it will not be the originator of a "good." Any good associated with government is the result of either a regulatory limitation on government, a reaction to demands of citizenry (which is its proper function), or the negation of some previous government action.

In the case of slavery in the West, it took two-and-a-half centuries for civil liberties to evolve to the point that the common citizenry, mostly non-voters, could organize popular antislavery associations with sufficient political power to begin to influence government action. Thus, the 1833 action that outlawed slavery in the United Kingdom did not represent a parliamentary epiphany. It was instead a reaction to the demands of the citizenry. In the same sense, the Emancipation Proclamation of 1863 and the Civil Rights Act of 1964 were governmental "goods," but they were reactions to demands of citizens and corrections of earlier bad governmental policies, both federal and state. But should political leadership declare it plans to initiate a helpful new program, one without precedent, watch out.   The intent may be good, but the consequences will almost always be bad, usually because it motives are selfish and will increase government influence and thereby power.

For slavery, that regression of Western governments from interference with natural rights of citizens finally came about when the 16th C Reformation in Europe led to 17C parliaments that began to cede natural rights in the 18th C to common citizens, permitting them to grapple with, and then abolish, that immorality. In medicine it had been the published findings of unprivileged physicians such as Morgagni (1761, well-to-do but raised by his mother), Auenbrugger (1761, son of an innkeeper), Gordon (1795, son of a tenant farmer), and Laennec (1819, son of a lawyer) that opened the 19th C golden age of medical progress.   In abolitionism it was writings of the unprivileged Nonconformists such as Sharp (1769, son of a senior Anglican cleric), Ramsay (1784, son of a ship's carpenter), Wilberforce (1787, son of a merchant), and Roscoe (1788, son of a market-gardener) that would lead to the 19th C abolition of slavery. Those at the top of the social order, the canonizers of the political hierarchy, whatever their personal opinion, were removed from the theater of autonomous action and therefore incapable of formulating *per se* practical solutions.

---

[21] Here it might be argued that it would have taken the industrial revolution in the United Kingdom (roughly dated from 1760 to 1840) time to develop to the point that human labor requirements decreased and abolition could be discontinued because its usefulness was ceasing. But the simultaneous reality of medical progress and moral abolition may not have been a coincidence. Both emerged from the general citizenry of Western nations, and both became possible with the protection of natural rights. Thus, by time, means, locus, and focus I argue the two events were part of a larger process released when the Reformation inspired civil liberties, and that process was a manifestation of the Judeo-Christian civilization, both a long time coming.

The Isagorial Theory of Human Progress states that the source of all *apolitical* human progress, as gauged by medical practice, is the collegial association of autonomous individuals with special or focused knowledge in the general population sharing a common interest and having a goal of self-betterment.[22] These associations in medicine were composed of practitioners who actually saw their patients and assumed the responsibility for their care. In abolitionism, moral leadership came not from the political or academic hierarchy. It came from citizens from all walks of life who viewed slavery as an affront to natural law and natural rights granted by God, rights they now had to a degree that permitted argument without fear of punishment from government. Addressed by religious associations, the moral force they recognized was based on autonomous "self-betterment" being denied to the enslaved. By becoming a potent political force they successfully caused government to abolish slavery. It appears that the Isagorial Theory of Human Progress applies to *political* progress as well as the apolitical.

THE END

---

[22] See Excursus 12 for more on the *Isagorial Theory of Human Progress.*

INDEX

CPSIA information can be obtained
at www.ICGtesting.com
Printed in the USA
LVHW051512310323
743145LV00007B/1045

9 781662 870859